The **BRUX** Method:

A neuroscience-based framework for relieving bruxism

Title: The BRUX Method
Subtitle: A neuroscience-based framework for relieving bruxism

Author: Randy Clare

Published by: Randy Clare
United States of America

ISBN

Paperback ISBN: 979-8-9949016-2-5

Printing Information

Printed in the United States of America
First Edition

For my wife Kerry, whose creativity sharpens every idea and whose belief in me never wavers. This book exists because you never let me stand still.

Table of Content

Introduction..8

Part I: Build: Making the Invisible Visible 21

Chapter 1: When the Body Bites Back 24

Chapter 2: Introducing the BRUX Method..............................41

Chapter 3: The power of noticing 55

Chapter 4: Mapping Your Jaw Habit 65

Part II: Relax Retraining the Reflex..............................75

Chapter 5: Relaxed Jaw Reset 78

Chapter 6: Breathing as Feedback 90

Chapter 7: Softening the Signal 108

Part III: Understand: Decoding Your Triggers 122

Chapter 8: Stress, Screens, and Cognitive Load 125

Chapter 9: Posture, Pressure and the Jaw..............................143

Chapter 10: Sleep, Light, and Sleep Clenching 156

Chapter 11: Hormones, Hydration, and Muscle Tone 173

Chapter 12: Pain, Protection, and the Nervous System..............................186

Chapter 13: Emotion, Control, and Holding On..............................200

Chapter 14: From Habit to Harmony 215

Chapter 15: Designing Daily Rituals 232

Chapter 16: The Body as Ongoing Feedback 244

Epilogue: Awareness Is Medicine, and BRUX Is the Way You Practice It 256

Acknowledgments..............................262

Preface

Why I Stopped Fighting My Jaw

For most of my professional life, I worked around bruxism without fully understanding the mechanics of the condition. My career has been rooted in dental devices. I spent years involved in solutions for snoring and sleep apnea, along with mouthguards and functional appliances designed to protect teeth, reduce clenching force, or reposition the jaw to relieve TMJ pain.

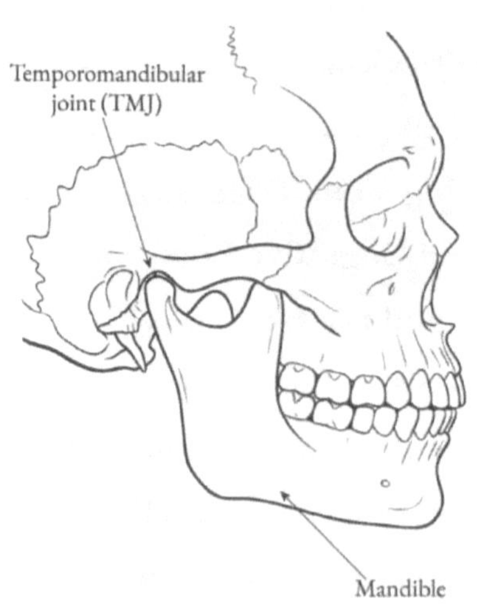

These devices serve an important purpose. They protect enamel. They reduce damage. They help people get through the night.

What they do not do is explain why the jaw keeps clenching in the first place. That question stayed in the background for a long time, even as my own body was giving me signals, I could no longer ignore. I have been a clencher and grinder for as long as I can remember. My awareness came slowly. Teeth that chipped too easily. Cracks that appeared without obvious cause.

At a dental meeting one year, a close friend and mentor, Dr. John Viviano from Toronto, looked at my teeth and asked a simple question. "What happened to your teeth?"

I did not have a good answer.

Not long after that, I woke up with severe pain in my temporomandibular joints (TMJ). It was unmistakable. I was in the middle of an acute TMJ episode. The pain was intense and persistent, lasting nearly a week. I understood what was happening and managed the episode, but something shifted for me. This was no longer theoretical. My jaw was demanding attention.

Over time, I invested heavily in restoring my smile. I spent close to thirty thousand dollars on dental work to repair the damage, some visible some invisible. My teeth looked better, but the clenching and grinding never stopped. I noticed something else. Whenever I was stressed or deeply focused, my jaw was clenched. I rarely noticed it in the moment. Awareness only arrived after the muscles were sore or the tension became overwhelming.

That disconnect became the turning point for the way I saw bruxism and resulted in a change in the way I approached my career. I stopped asking how to fight the clenching and started asking why it was happening at all. In the last several years, I have dedicated myself to understanding bruxism at its source. Modern neurobiology does not view bruxism as a bad habit or a simple dental problem.

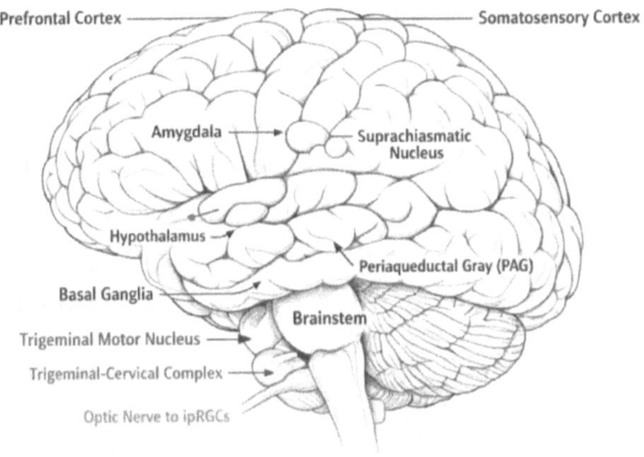

This is not my brain…. The labels are areas of the brain that are involved in bruxism It understands it as a somatic expression of the autonomic nervous system, specifically an extension of the fight or flight response.

When the brain perceives a threat, whether physical or psychological, it activates a cascade designed to prepare the body for action. Hormones surge. Heart rate increases. Muscles brace.

The trigeminal nerve, which controls the jaw closing muscles, is directly involved in this response. In primitive survival contexts, clenching the jaw stabilizes the head and prepares the body for defense.

In modern life, the threats rarely resolve. Deadlines at work, computer and phone screens, responsibility, and constant stimulation keep the nervous system activated without providing a physical outlet. The energy has nowhere to go. It becomes trapped as muscle tension. For many people, the jaw becomes the default storehouse for tension. This reframing changed how I saw my own clenching. It was not a flaw. It was information.

Once I understood bruxism as a nervous system reflex rather than a failure of discipline, awareness became the logical starting point for change. You cannot interrupt a reflex you do not know is happening. You cannot choose differently if the behavior never reaches consciousness.

That is where awareness becomes active rather than passive. In the context of bruxism, awareness is not a byproduct of treatment. It is the treatment. Traditional night guards act like helmets. They protect teeth from damage but allow the battle to continue.

Biofeedback, when used properly, acts more like a negotiator. It brings unconscious behavior into conscious awareness at the exact moment it begins.

Over time, that awareness changes the habit itself.

By repeatedly noticing the first signs of clenching, pressure, breath holding, or facial tension, the nervous system learns a new baseline. Reflex becomes choice. Choice becomes habit. The jaw begins to rest in a state of safety rather than vigilance. Lips together. Teeth apart. Tongue supported. Breathing steady.

This book exists because too many people are suffering from the effects of uncontrolled bruxism without understanding what their bodies are trying to do. They protect their teeth while their nervous systems remain on high alert. They are told to relax without being shown how. They are left managing symptoms instead of learning skills.

The BRUX Method is my attempt to change that.

It brings together habit science, neurobiology, lived experience, and practical tools into a process that people can use. Not to force the jaw into submission, but to teach the body that it no longer needs to brace. If you are holding this book because your teeth are wearing down, your jaw hurts, or your headaches will not let you ignore them anymore, you are not broken. Your nervous system has learned a pattern that once made sense. This book will help you learn a new one.

Randy Clare

Introduction
The Unseen Habit Shaping Your Days

Most people do not decide to clench their jaw.

They discover it in the aftermath. A headache that greets them before coffee. Teeth that suddenly feel fragile. A chipped edge that makes no sense. A sore jaw that shows up after a long day of "just working."

Sometimes the first clue is a comment from a dentist. Sometimes it is a bed partner who hears grinding at night. Often, it is a slow accumulation of symptoms that never quite add up.

If that is you, I want to start with a simple reassurance.

This is not a character flaw. It is not a lack of discipline. It is not proof that you are doing life wrong.

Bruxism is best understood as an unconscious pattern that lives below deliberate choice.[1] It is a body-level response that can become a default behavior.[9] Once you see it that way, the problem becomes clearer and the path forward becomes practical. This book exists to make that path real.

Why Do So Many People Clench Without Realizing It?

People often assume that if they are doing something harmful, they would notice. Bruxism breaks that assumption. Clenching and grinding are largely driven by the autonomic nervous system,[7] the system that regulates survival functions such as arousal, vigilance, heart rate, and recovery.[19] Much of that activity is managed outside conscious awareness. Your brain does not ask permission to tighten your jaw any more than it asks permission to speed up your pulse during stress.

That is not a defect. It is efficiency.

The nervous system is designed to protect you. When it senses threat, pressure, urgency, or overload, it prepares the body for action. The jaw is part of that preparation.

The jaw closing muscles are powerful and stabilizing. They help brace the head and neck. They also express strain, restraint, and internal effort. This is why bruxism often shows up in three predictable places. First, it appears during stress, anger, urgency, or emotional suppression. The jaw becomes the place where the body "holds it together." Second, it appears during concentration. Many people clench while reading, emailing, driving, lifting, or thinking hard.[15] The brain narrows focus and filters internal sensation. The job gets done. The jaw pays the price.

Third, it appears during sleep. Sleep Bruxism often occurs during brief shifts in arousal, when the brain transitions between sleep stages.[6] These events can be too short to form memory.[8] You wake up with the consequences and no recollection of the action.

The pattern is consistent. Symptoms show up before awareness because the behavior is running in the background. If you have ever thought, "I would stop if I knew I was doing it," you are not wrong. You simply have not been given a reliable way to know.

What Bruxism Really Is

Bruxism is not only "teeth grinding."[2] That is the common shorthand, but it misses a large portion of what people do. Clinically, bruxism is repetitive jaw muscle activity that can include clenching, grinding, bracing, or thrusting of the jaw.[3]

That matters because many people do not grind loudly. They brace. They press. They hold. Their teeth may touch lightly for long periods.

9

Their jaw may stay rigid even with little tooth contact. They may wake with pain despite minimal wear.

Modern clinical thinking also distinguishes between two forms.[1] Awake Bruxism (AB) is usually tied to habit, stress, concentration, and emotional load. Sleep Bruxism (SB) is tied to sleep-related arousal and nervous system activity during sleep. These forms overlap, but they are not identical. The difference matters because the tools for change are not the same.

You will learn both in this book, and you will learn how to tell which pattern is driving your symptoms.

Why Clenching Persists Even When Pain Is Treated

Many people treat the pain and assume the habit will stop. Sometimes it does, briefly. Often it does not. That can feel discouraging. It can also feel confusing. If the jaw no longer hurts, why does it still clench? The simplest answer is this. Pain is a symptom. Bruxism is a learned pattern.[9]

When bruxism has been repeated for years, the nervous system begins to treat it as a default.[10] The body learns that clenching equals readiness. It becomes a background setting. Even if you reduce pain with medication, therapy, massage, or dental treatment, the underlying "clench command" may still be running. This is why purely passive solutions often disappoint people.

Night guards and appliances are important for protection. They reduce damage to teeth and joints. They can reduce friction and distribute force. They can improve comfort. But protection does not automatically change the brain's habit loop.[11] In other words, you can wear your plastic night guard every night and still be grinding.

This is not a criticism of dental protection. It is a clarification of its role. Protection is often necessary. It is rarely sufficient.[12]

If you want the clenching itself to change, you must work with the system that produces it. That system is the nervous system. That is where habit science becomes useful.

How Habit Science Changes the Way We Approach Bruxism

Habit science gives us a better question. Instead of asking, "How do I stop clenching?" we ask, "What is the loop that keeps clenching going?"

Every habit loop has three parts.[15,16]

A cue or trigger that starts the pattern.

A response that the body performs.
A reinforcement that teaches the brain to keep using the response.

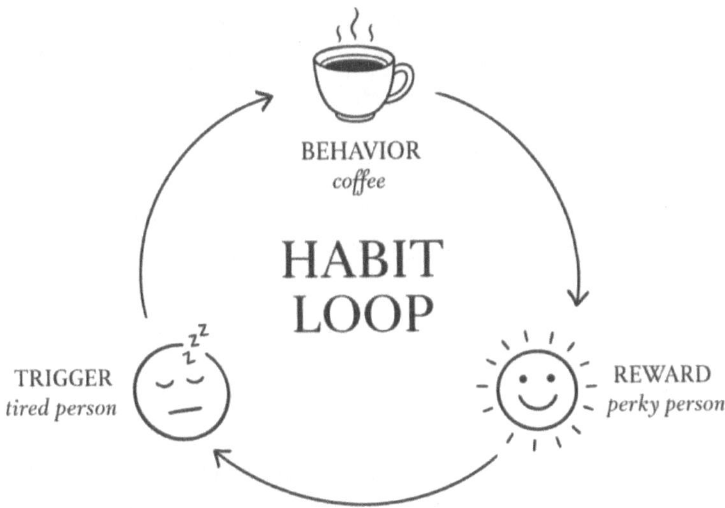

In bruxism, the trigger is often stress, concentration, micro-arousals in sleep, or sensory overload. The response is jaw muscle activation. The reinforcement is not always obvious, but it is real.

In some cases, clenching creates a brief sense of stability, control, or readiness. In other cases, it may change arousal level in a way that the nervous system learns as regulation. Even if the outcome is harmful long-term, the brain learns that the action serves a purpose in the moment.

That is why bruxism persists.

The good news is that habit loops can be changed. [16] Not by force. Not by self-judgment. Not by pretending you are relaxed. They change through awareness, interruption, and replacement. The nervous system learns through repetition. It learns what you practice.

This is the foundation of the BRUX Method.

What This Book Will Help You Do Differently

If you have been stuck in the cycle of "symptoms, treatment, relapse," the BRUX Method will help you shift from passive protection to active retraining.

You will learn how to:

1) Identify the pattern earlier—You will learn how to notice clenching before it becomes pain. You will learn the early signals that usually arrive first, such as breath holding, facial tension, tongue pressure, and jaw bracing.

2) Understand your triggers without blaming yourself —You will learn how to map the situations and states that provoke clenching. This includes stress, focus, posture, sleep disruption, light exposure, and emotional suppression. You will learn to treat triggers as information, not evidence of weakness.

3) Interrupt the loop in real time — You will learn practical interventions that are small enough to use during real life, not only during quiet moments. The goal is not to be perfect. The goal is to become responsive.

4) Replace clenching with a stable baseline — You will learn the resting pattern that supports a calm nervous system. Lips together. Teeth apart. Tongue supported. Breath steady. This is not a slogan. It is a physical signature of safety.

5) Sustain change through habit stacking and daily rhythm — You will build routines that reduce relapse risk and help your body default to ease. You will learn how to design a day that does not constantly recruit the jaw as a coping mechanism.

This book does not ask you to become a different person. It asks you to become more aware of what your body is already doing, and more skilled in how you respond.

Why Awareness Is the Beginning of Relief

Awareness is often misunderstood as passive noticing.

In bruxism recovery, awareness is an active mechanism. It changes what is possible in the moment. If clenching is unconscious, you cannot choose differently.[17] The loop runs. The body braces. The damage accumulates.

When awareness is introduced, you gain a point of leverage.[15,17] The moment you notice, you interrupt automaticity. You move activity from reflex to choice, even if the choice is small at first.

This is also where biofeedback can help. Biofeedback is not a cure, and it is not required to benefit from this book. It is a tool that accelerates learning for some people by making the invisible visible.[13] A simple signal, such as vibration, can bring a clench into awareness in real time.

Over repeated use, the brain begins to recognize the sensation that precedes the signal. The skill becomes internal. The device becomes less necessary.[14] Whether you use a tool or train awareness manually, the principle is the same. Awareness is how the nervous system updates its defaults.

Why This Book Exists

The BRUX Method began in the intersection of behavioral science, clinical dentistry, and stress physiology. It also began in stories like Sarah's. People who woke up sore, foggy, and frustrated. People who tried mouthguards, Botox, massage, meditation, and still clenched. People who were told it was "just stress" without being given a process.

They did not need another vague instruction to relax. They needed a framework. They needed skills. They needed a way to practice change in the moments that matter, which are often small and frequent. They needed a way to stop treating bruxism as a mystery and start treating it as a learnable pattern. That is what this book provides.

How to Use This Book

This book is organized into five parts. Each part builds on the last.

Part I, Build – You will learn where your tension hides, how it shows up, and how to map your personal pattern without judgment.

Part II, Relax – You will learn regulation tools that reduce the body's need to brace. Breath, posture, sensory calming, and release strategies are introduced as skills, not advice.

Part III, Understand – You will explore deeper drivers such as screens, sleep disruption, light, posture, and cognitive load. You will connect science to sensation.

14

Part IV, Restore – You will learn how biology influences muscle tone and resilience. Hydration, hormones, pain pathways, and nervous system protection patterns are addressed in practical terms.

Part V, Exchange – You will integrate everything into daily rhythm and habit stacking. You will learn how to sustain change, reframe relapse, and build trust in your body long-term.

Each section follows a consistent rhythm: a story to ground the experience, the science that explains it, practices you can use immediately, reflection prompts, and an integration tip to help your nervous system learn through repetition.

You can read straight through, or you can start where you feel the most pain and return to earlier chapters later. If you are overwhelmed, begin with one practice and repeat it daily. Skill builds faster through repetition than through intensity.

The Habit Beneath the Habit

Bruxism is rarely just a "teeth problem." Teeth are where the evidence shows up, but the behavior often lives deeper in the nervous system. At its core, clenching is frequently a strategy for control and safety,[18,19] even when you do not consciously choose it. When life feels fast, uncertain, emotionally charged, or relentlessly demanding, the body looks for something it can stabilize. The jaw is an obvious candidate. It is strong. It is designed to generate force. It sits close to the brain and shares circuitry with systems that manage vigilance, threat detection, and motor readiness.

When pressure rises, the jaw becomes a convenient place for the nervous system to concentrate effort. It can tighten quickly, hold tension for long periods, and create a temporary feeling of containment. That is why many people clench during moments that do not seem dramatic. A difficult email. A complex decision. A

15

conversation where they are biting back words. A day that requires constant competence.

The jaw becomes the body's way of saying, "I have to stay ready," even when the true demand is emotional, cognitive, or relational rather than physical. This is not weakness. It is endurance. Most chronic clenchers are not fragile people. They are often capable, conscientious, and highly responsible. They push through fatigue. They stay composed. They delay their needs. Over time, the jaw learns to participate in that lifestyle. It becomes part of the holding pattern. It tightens when you concentrate. It braces when you try to stay calm. It locks when you carry more than you can metabolize.

If you have been clenching for years, the habit may feel personal, as if your body is stubborn or defective. It is not. Your nervous system adopted a strategy that worked well enough to get you through. The problem is that what works in the short term becomes costly when it becomes chronic. A protective reflex turns into a default setting. Muscle tone rises. Pain sensitivity increases. Sleep becomes more fragile.

The jaw keeps doing its job because no one has told it, in a language the nervous system trusts, that the danger has passed. This book is an invitation to reverse that training.

The work is not to force your body into perfect relaxation. The work is to teach safety in small, repeatable ways. Softness is not surrender. Rest is not laziness. Releasing the jaw is not giving up. It is a skillful update to your nervous system's threat model. It is the moment you stop asking your jaw to carry what your life is asking of you.

Each time you notice tightening and choose a different response, you create a new association. Awareness becomes the cue. Regulation becomes the response. Safety becomes the reward. Over time, the old pattern loses urgency. The new pattern becomes easier to access under pressure.

That is the real shift. You move from bracing by default to responding with intention. You stop treating clenching as a character flaw and start treating it as information. And you build a relationship with your body that is based on listening, adjustment, and recovery rather than criticism and control.

That is the work.
That is the BRUX Method.

Pause and Practice

One-Minute Baseline Check

Do this once right now.

Let your lips come together gently.

Separate your teeth slightly.

Place the tongue lightly on the roof of the mouth, just behind your front teeth. (whisper the word "with" to find the spot)

Exhale slowly through the nose.

Ask one question: "What is my jaw doing right now?"

Do not force anything. Do not judge the answer. Just notice.

That is your first rep.

References

Bruxism Definition, Classification, and Physiology

1. Lobbezoo F, Ahlberg J, Raphael KG, et al. International consensus on the assessment of bruxism: Report of a work in progress. J Oral Rehabil. 2018;45(11):837-844. doi:10.1111/joor.12663

2. Lobbezoo F, Zaag J van der, Naeije M. Bruxism: Its multiple causes and its effects on dental implants – an updated review. J Oral Rehabil. 2006;33(4):293-300. doi:10.1111/j.1365-2842.2006.01627.x

3. Manfredini D, Serra-Negra J, Carboncini F, Lobbezoo F. Current concepts of bruxism. Int J Prosthodont. 2017;30(5):437-438. doi:10.11607/ijp.5210

Awake vs Sleep Bruxism

4. Manfredini D, Lobbezoo F. Relationship between bruxism and temporomandibular disorders: A systematic review of literature from 1998 to 2008. Oral Surg Oral Med Oral Pathol Oral Radiol Endod. 2010;109(6):e26-e50. doi:10.1016/j.tripleo.2010.02.013
5. Lobbezoo F, Aarab G, Wetselaar P, et al. Tooth wear and bruxism: A critical review. J Oral Rehabil. 2013;40(2):124-134. doi:10.1111/joor.12010

Sleep Bruxism, Arousals, and Autonomic Activity

6. Kato T, Thie NMR, Montplaisir JY, Lavigne GJ. Bruxism and orofacial movements during sleep. Dent Clin North Am. 2001;45(4):657-684.

7. Lavigne GJ, Kato T, Kolta A, Sessle BJ. Neurobiological mechanisms involved in sleep bruxism. Crit Rev Oral Biol Med. 2003;14(1):30-46. doi:10.1177/154411130301400104

8. Huynh N, Kato T, Rompré PH, et al. Sleep bruxism is associated with micro-arousals and an increase in cardiac sympathetic activity. J Sleep Res. 2006;15(3):339-346. doi:10.1111/j.1365-2869.2006.00536.x

Pain vs Habit Persistence

9. Raphael KG, Santiago V, Lobbezoo F. Is bruxism a disorder or a behavior? Rethinking the international consensus on bruxism. J Oral Rehabil. 2016;43(10):791-798. doi:10.1111/joor.12413

10. Svensson P, Jadidi F, Arima T, Baad-Hansen L, Sessle BJ. Relationships between craniofacial pain and bruxism. J Oral Rehabil. 2008;35(7):524-547. doi:10.1111/j.1365-2842.2008.01852.x

Oral Appliances as Protection, Not Habit Change

11. Okeson JP. Management of temporomandibular disorders and occlusion. 8th ed. St Louis, MO: Elsevier; 2020.

12. American Academy of Sleep Medicine. Clinical practice guideline for the treatment of bruxism and sleep-related movement disorders. J Clin Sleep Med. 2018;14(9):1561-1567.

Biofeedback and Behavioral Interventions

13. Jadidi F, Castrillon E, Svensson P. Effect of biofeedback on awake bruxism behavior: A randomized controlled trial. J Oral Rehabil. 2013;40(8):590-597. doi:10.1111/joor.12069

14. Watanabe T, Ichikawa K, Clark GT. Behavioral management of awake bruxism. J Oral Facial Pain Headache. 2015;29(4):341-349. doi:10.11607/ofph.1448

Habit Science and Automaticity

15. Wood W, Rünger D. Psychology of habit. Annu Rev Psychol. 2016;67:289-314. doi:10.1146/annurev-psych-122414-033417

16. Duhigg C. The Power of Habit. New York, NY: Random House; 2012.

17. Clear J. Atomic Habits. New York, NY: Avery; 2018.

Nervous System Regulation and Threat Processing

18. Porges SW. The polyvagal theory: New insights into adaptive reactions of the autonomic nervous system. Cleve Clin J Med. 2009;76(Suppl 2):S86-S90. doi:10.3949/ccjm.76.s2.17
19. McEwen BS. Stress, adaptation, and disease: Allostasis and allostatic load. Ann N Y Acad Sci. 1998;840:33-44. doi:10.1111/j.1749-6632.1998.tb09546.x

Part I: Build: Making the Invisible Visible

Learn how to recognize your unique tension patterns and transform them into useful information.

Meet Sarah. Sarah is 37, a designer with a mind that never really powers down. Her days are spent at a laptop, shoulders slightly raised, chin forward, eyes narrowed in focus. At night she tries to rest, but she keeps half-scrolling, half-sleeping, as if her nervous system does not know how to downshift.

For months she has carried symptoms that feel unrelated: shoulder pain, fatigue that lingers behind her eyes, and headaches that flare without warning and spread across her temples. She assumes it is posture, stress, caffeine, or a bad pillow.

She starts building her life around the discomfort, choosing quieter plans, avoiding long drives, rationing energy like it is a limited resource.

She becomes a collector of fixes. An ergonomic chair. New pillows. More water. Less coffee. Ibuprofen in every bag.

She stretches her neck in the shower and rolls her shoulders at stoplights. Nothing changes. The unpredictability is the worst part. It makes her cautious. She hesitates before committing to weekends.

She loses patience in meetings, not because she is difficult, but because she can feel pressure building and wants to escape before it becomes a headache. Quietly, she starts to wonder if this is simply her normal now.

At a routine dental visit, her dentist pauses longer than usual. He points out tiny cracks and flattened enamel on her teeth.

"Do you clench your teeth?" he asks. Sarah laughs. "No, I don't think so." It feels honest. She would notice clenching, wouldn't she? He nods. "Most people don't know they do. It's often unconscious.

The jaw braces when the nervous system is under load, especially during intense focus or sleep."

On the drive home, the scattered pieces finally connect. The breath she holds when she concentrates. The way her teeth touch when she is deep in a project. The tight face in the morning and the pain in her face by afternoon.

Bruxism is not just grinding. It is bracing and holding, a reflex the body uses to create stability under pressure. And like any chronic condition, it has been shaping how she lives, chooses, and interacts with the world.

For the first time in months, she feels something steadier than hope. Not a promise of an instant fix, but the relief of an explanation. If the habit is unconscious, it can be made visible. If it can be made visible, it can change.

Chapter 1: When the Body Bites Back

Jaw tension rarely starts as a jaw problem. For most people, it reflects how the nervous system conserves effort by automating protective responses.[1] When pressure rises, the brain stabilizes the body without conscious permission, recruiting structures like the jaw that provide rapid mechanical support.[4,2]

That is why bruxism often feels confusing. You experience the consequences, but not the cause.

The BRUX Method exists to solve that mismatch. It is built on a simple premise: jaw clenching is not primarily a dental issue. It is a nervous system behavior that becomes a habit. And habits are changeable when you apply the right leverage.

This book will not ask you to "try harder" to relax. It will teach you how to change the conditions that make your nervous system default to bracing, then install a new default that is easier to maintain than clenching.

What Bruxism Is, Clinically and Functionally

Bruxism is often reduced to "teeth grinding," but modern clinical definitions are broader and more accurate. Bruxism is repetitive jaw muscle activity that can include clenching, grinding, bracing, and jaw thrusting.[2] Many people never grind audibly. They hold tension. They compress the bite. They brace without movement.

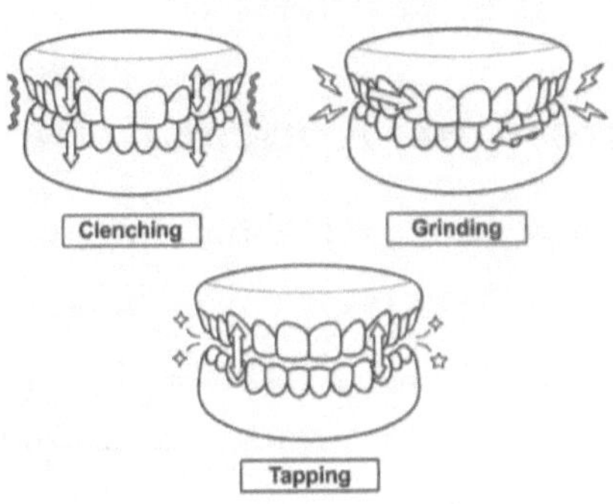

Clinicians distinguish two forms based on when they occur:

Sleep bruxism is nocturnal and commonly occurs during brief arousal shifts in sleep. As the brain transitions through lighter sleep and micro-arousals, short bursts of jaw muscle activity can appear. These events are closely linked to arousal physiology and autonomic activation, and some researchers have proposed broader protective roles during sleep, although the exact biological function is still being studied.[4,7]

Awake bruxism happens during the day, when focus or frustration sneaks into muscle tone. Maybe you're driving in traffic, scrolling through news, or chasing a deadline. You notice your shoulders are high, your breath shallow, and if you paid attention, your jaw would likely be engaged, and your teeth will be touching too.

These categories matter because they imply different mechanisms. Sleep bruxism is often tied to arousal physiology and sleep fragmentation, and may co-occur with factors that influence airway stability, although the relationships are not fully causal or uniform across individuals. [4,7]

Awake bruxism is often tied to threat processing, attention, and learned habit loops during focused tasks. Both forms share a core theme: jaw activity is driven by nervous system state, not by a lack of discipline.

Why Symptoms Appear Before Awareness

The most important fact about bruxism is that it is frequently unconscious.

The brain is hierarchical. High level regions handle planning and conscious control. Lower regions handle survival, reflexes, and repetitive behaviors.

Bruxism is often expressed through motor and arousal systems that operate largely outside conscious awareness. Research links sleep bruxism in particular to arousal-related physiology, and awake bruxism to learned behavior patterns that can become automatic with repetition.[4,7,13,14]

This creates a predictable delay:

The jaw can be active for years without awareness because the behavior is treated as "normal" by the system that generates it. The damage accumulates slowly. Enamel has no nerves. Muscles adapt. Your body can run a high load pattern quietly until it crosses a threshold.

Sleep makes the awareness gap larger. Most jaw events occur during brief arousals that you do not remember. The result is morning symptoms with no clear story. The BRUX Method begins by closing this gap. You cannot change what you cannot detect. Awareness is not a motivational concept. It is a neurological mechanism that turns an automatic loop into a modifiable one.

The Mechanics of Damage

Tooth Wear and Micro-Fractures

When upper and lower teeth repeatedly meet under elevated force, the risk of mechanical wear and micro-damage increases over time. Enamel is highly durable, but it is not designed for prolonged, repeated loading outside normal chewing patterns.[10] It's built to withstand the pressure of chewing for a few seconds at a time, not hours of unconscious clenching.

In early stages, subtle wear facets or micro-damage may develop that you may not notice day to day. In some cases, a dentist can detect early signs such as wear patterns, small chips, or stress-related changes during an exam.[10]

Over months or years, these fissures deepen, spreading like hairline fractures in glass. The enamel thins, exposing the softer dentin beneath, a material more porous and sensitive to temperature and touch. That's when you start noticing twinges from cold drinks or aching after meals.

Once enamel is lost, it doesn't regenerate. The body can heal bone and skin, but not the structure of enamel. If excessive forces persist without intervention, cumulative changes can include flattened cusps, chipped restorations, shortened tooth structure, and functional bite changes in susceptible individuals.[10]

Clenching and grinding are not simply 'bad habits.' They can act as repeated mechanical loading that teeth and restorations may tolerate for a time, but that can increase the likelihood of damage when the pattern is frequent or forceful. [10]

The earlier you recognize it, the easier it is to intervene, not just with dental repair, but with awareness. Because what wears down your teeth isn't weakness; it's repetition. And repetition, once seen, can be retrained.

27

Joint Stress

Your temporomandibular joint (TMJ) is one of the most complex joints in the human body, a tiny hinge-and-slide mechanism that lets your jaw open, close, and glide forward or sideways with remarkable precision. But like any hinge, it depends on balance. When that balance is lost through constant clenching, strain begins to build.

Each episode of bruxism compresses the joint capsule and the small disc that cushions movement between the jawbone and skull. Over time, this pressure irritates the surrounding ligaments and muscles, creating inflammation and micro-swelling. You might notice subtle clicking or popping when you yawn or chew, or a sense of fullness and pressure near the ears.

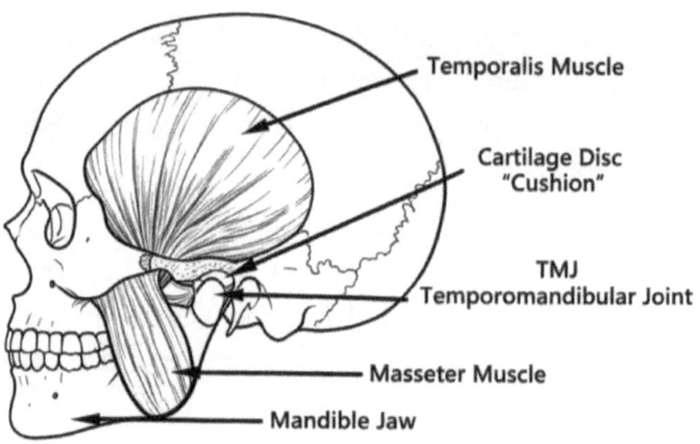

Clicking, popping, or a sense of pressure near the ears can reflect altered joint mechanics or changes in how the disc and joint surfaces move, although these signs are not diagnostic on their own. In some individuals, sustained overloading is associated with joint irritation and, in more advanced cases, structural changes that may be evaluated with imaging when clinically indicated.[10,11]

TMJ stress isn't just mechanical; it's systemic. When the joint is inflamed, nearby muscles stay tense to guard it, perpetuating the cycle of tightness. Breaking that loop begins with gentleness unclenching the jaw, spacing the teeth slightly, and allowing the system to rest. Relief isn't only about reducing pain; it's about restoring the natural rhythm between protection and release.

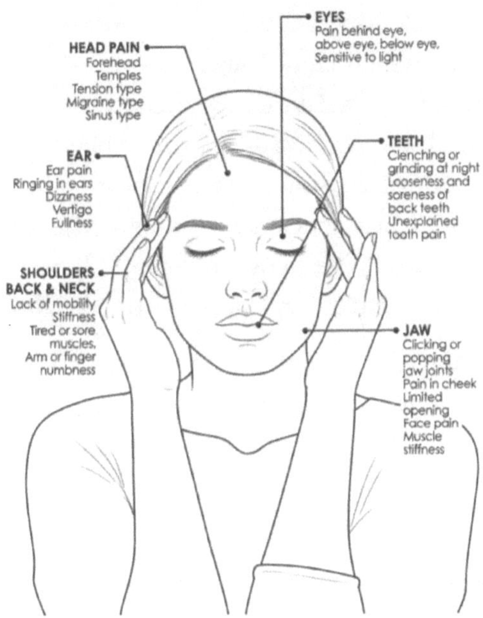

Headaches and Referred Pain

Jaw pain rarely stays in the jaw.

The masseter and temporalis muscles, which drive clenching and grinding, share nerve pathways with areas of the head, temples, and even around the eyes. Because of these shared circuits, the brain can misinterpret where pain begins, a phenomenon called referred pain.

29

That's why jaw tension can present as head, temple, or facial pain that resembles tension-type headache patterns, and may coexist with other headache disorders.[9] You might feel a dull ache behind your eyes, a band-like pressure around your forehead, or pain that seems to pulse from your temples. It's easy to treat the symptoms, painkillers, caffeine, or rest, without realizing the true source is the jaw's relentless workload.

Chronic muscle overactivity can contribute to local fatigue and sensitization, which may lower the threshold for discomfort over time and make normal activities such as chewing feel more irritating.[9] A normal bite or even gentle chewing can begin to feel uncomfortable. Releasing jaw tension often brings surprising relief to the head and face because it quiets the overactive neural web connecting them. When you unclench, blood flow improves, oxygen returns to the muscles, and nerve endings calm down.

Your jaw and your head are in constant conversation. When one relaxes, the other follows. Understanding that link turns pain from a mystery into a message one you can finally answer with awareness instead of endurance.

Neck and Shoulder Strain

The jaw doesn't work alone; it's part of a muscular team that includes the neck and shoulders.

When your jaw muscles engage, the stabilizing muscles of the upper body, like the trapezius and sternocleidomastoid, often contract in sync, forming what's known as a bracing pattern.

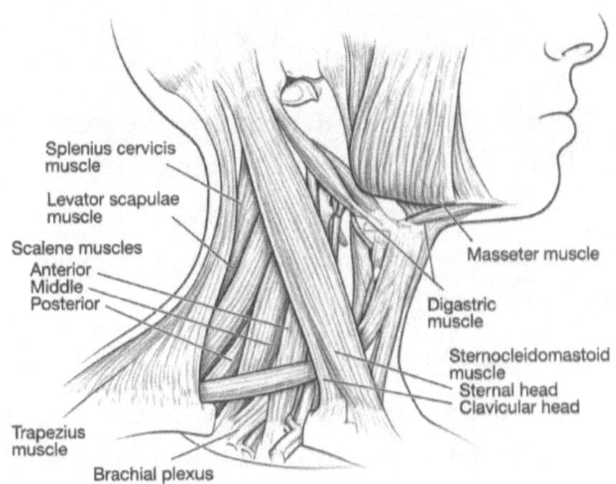

It's your body's way of steadying the scaffold. When the jaw clenches, the head subtly shifts forward, and the neck muscles engage to hold it there. The shoulders follow, creeping upward toward the ears. This alignment, repeated daily, changes posture over time tightening fascia and compressing joints in the cervical spine.

Electromyography studies demonstrate that jaw, neck, and shoulder muscles can co-activate during stress and sustained mental effort, consistent with a broader bracing pattern. Many people notice that when they reduce jaw tension, their shoulders and neck also soften, reflecting how closely these systems coordinate under load.[12]

Over time, these coupled contractions create a chain of tension that radiates downward: headaches, neck stiffness, and upper back soreness that no massage seems to fix for long. The relief fades because the root isn't in the shoulders it's in the jaw's unconscious command.

Learning to relax the jaw, to create space between the teeth, doesn't just protect oral structures it resets posture. When the jaw releases, the entire upper body follows, reminding you that tension is never local. It's a full-body language waiting to be translated.

Sleep Disturbance and Fatigue

Bruxism doesn't clock out at bedtime. For many, it becomes most active in sleep, especially during micro-arousals, brief awakenings when the brain shifts between light and deep sleep. Each jaw contraction pulls the body closer to wakefulness, spiking heart rate and disrupting the continuity of rest.

You might not remember waking, but your body does. Nighttime jaw activity often clusters around micro-arousals and is associated with sympathetic activation and more fragmented sleep. This can reduce the perceived restorative quality of sleep, even when total sleep time looks adequate. [4,6,7] The next day, you feel foggy, drained, or irritable, symptoms nearly identical to insomnia.

This disruption is self-perpetuating. Poor sleep heightens stress sensitivity, which increases jaw activity the following night. The cycle repeats until exhaustion feels normal. For many, this pattern goes unnoticed for years, misattributed to "poor sleep hygiene" or general anxiety.

Behavioral and biofeedback-based approaches can improve awareness and reduce jaw-muscle overactivity in some individuals, particularly for awake bruxism. For sleep bruxism, these approaches may help indirectly by lowering overall arousal and improving pre-sleep regulation, although effects vary.[15,16] When the jaw learns safety while awake, it can carry that memory into sleep.

Fatigue isn't just about lost hours of rest; it's about a system that never fully powers down. Reclaiming that rest begins with what seems simplest: awareness, breath, and the courage to let go even in the dark.

Primary and Secondary Drivers

Not all bruxism has the same upstream cause. Some cases are considered primary and reflect learned patterns shaped by stress, attention, and nervous system state. Others are secondary and are influenced by factors such as medication effects, neurological conditions, or sleep disordered breathing and airway instability.

The BRUX Method does not ignore these distinctions. It simply starts from the most useful common denominator: regardless of origin, the jaw is responding to signals. When you reduce the signal and change the response, the output changes.

The BRUX Method as a Scientific Framework

BRUX is not a slogan. It is an applied model of behavior change rooted in neuroscience, physiology, and CBT principles.

B: Build Awareness—You develop real time detection of tension before it becomes pain. This can be done with interoceptive skill building and, when useful, objective cues such as biofeedback. The goal is to interrupt the habit loop early.

R: Relax the Response—You train the nervous system to downshift on demand. This is not passive relaxation. It is active regulation, often via breath, posture, and sensory safety signals that reduce motor drive to the jaw.

U: Understand Triggers—You identify the conditions that reliably pull you out of neutral. These triggers can be cognitive, emotional, postural, environmental, chemical, or sleep related. When you name triggers precisely, the problem becomes solvable.

X: Exchange the Pattern—You replace bracing with a new default that is easier to repeat than clenching. This includes mechanical changes, behavioral substitutions, and ritual design so the nervous system has a stable alternative under load.

The scientific logic is straightforward. Habits are not erased. They are overwritten. When you repeatedly pair a trigger with a new response and a new reward, your brain updates the prediction: bracing is no longer necessary for safety, focus, or control.

That is why awareness is medicine. The moment you notice tension; a different part of the brain comes online. Inhibition becomes possible. Choice becomes possible. Recovery begins.

Why Protection Alone Is Not Enough

Many people try to solve bruxism by protecting teeth. Protection can be appropriate, especially at night, but protection does not retrain the underlying loop. A guard can reduce damage while the nervous system continues to brace.

The BRUX Method uses protection when needed, but it prioritizes retraining. If you teach the system to regulate, you reduce the need for the jaw to "do a job" it was never meant to do.

The Real Goal of This Book

The goal is not perfect stillness. The goal is a nervous system that recovers quickly.

Your jaw is not betraying you. It is adapting to perceived demands. When you give the nervous system better tools, the jaw no longer needs to volunteer as the stabilizer of your entire life.

This chapter establishes the core promise: bruxism becomes manageable when you treat it as a nervous system habit with identifiable drivers, not as a mysterious flaw you must endure.

The Brux Method: A New Pathway for Calm

Bruxism often feels like a problem that appears out of nowhere, but it follows a predictable biological pattern. The nervous system is built for efficiency, and it automates protective responses to stress, focus, vigilance, and arousal.

One of the most common places the body recruits for this protection is the jaw, because the jaw is a powerful stabilizer within the craniomandibular system. As a result, many people experience headaches, facial fatigue, tooth sensitivity, and morning jaw stiffness long before they ever notice clenching.

Symptoms usually arrive before awareness because the behavior is generated by lower brain and brainstem circuits that manage reflexive motor patterns and habit loops without conscious oversight.

Clinically, bruxism is not simply "teeth grinding." It is repetitive jaw muscle activity that can include clenching, grinding, bracing, and jaw thrusting. Many people do not grind audibly at all. They brace and compress.

Bruxism is also divided into sleep bruxism and awake bruxism, which share overlapping features but are driven by different mechanisms. Sleep bruxism is classified as a sleep related movement disorder and is often associated with micro arousals that fragment sleep and trigger rhythmic jaw muscle bursts.

Awake bruxism is considered a daytime behavior pattern, often linked to cognitive load, emotional pressure, and sustained concentration. Both forms are strongly influenced by nervous system state, not by willpower.

This chapter establishes why jaw tension becomes more than a local issue. The muscles of mastication (chewing muscles) can transmit strain into the temples and head, contributing to tension type headaches.

The trigeminal nerve can amplify facial and head pain when muscle activity stays elevated. At night, repeated arousal spikes can erode restorative sleep, producing fatigue even when total sleep time seems adequate.

Bruxism can be primary, shaped by learned stress and habit responses, or secondary, influenced by factors like medications, neurological conditions, or sleep disordered breathing. Regardless of origin, the central insight remains the same: the jaw is responding to signals, not malfunctioning randomly.

This chapter introduces the BRUX Method as a science grounded framework for change.

Build Awareness closes the gap between cause and consequence so you can interrupt the loop early.

Relax the Response trains downshifting skills that reduce motor drive and protective bracing.

Understand Triggers identifies the specific cognitive, emotional, postural, chemical, and sleep related conditions that reliably provoke clenching.

Exchange the Pattern replaces bracing with a new default through repetition, behavior design, and supportive rituals. The method is based on the neuroscience of habit overwriting, not habit deletion.

New pathways become dominant when they are practiced consistently under real triggers.

Finally, the chapter clarifies the aim of the book. Success is not perfect stillness. Success is a nervous system that recovers quickly.

Protection alone may reduce damage, but it does not retrain the underlying pattern. Awareness does. The moment you notice tension, change has already begun, because noticing recruits higher regulatory circuits and makes a different response possible.

References

Bruxism Definition, Classification, and Conceptual Framework

1. Lobbezoo F, Ahlberg J, Glaros AG, et al. Bruxism defined and graded: an international consensus. J Oral Rehabil.2013;40(1):2-4. doi:10.1111/joor.12011

2. Lobbezoo F, Ahlberg J, Raphael KG, et al. International consensus on the assessment of bruxism: report of a work in progress. J Oral Rehabil. 2018;45(11):837-844. doi:10.1111/joor.12663

3. Verhoeff MC, Lobbezoo F, Ahlberg J, et al. Updating the bruxism definitions: report of an international consensus meeting. J Oral Rehabil. 2025;52(9):1335-1342. doi:10.1111/joor.13985

4. Raphael KG, Santiago V, Lobbezoo F. Is bruxism a disorder or a behavior? Rethinking the international consensus. J Oral Rehabil. 2016;43(10):791-798. doi:10.1111/joor.12413

Awake vs Sleep Bruxism

5. Manfredini D, Lobbezoo F. Relationship between bruxism and temporomandibular disorders: a systematic review of literature from 1998 to 2008. Oral Surg Oral Med Oral Pathol Oral Radiol Endod. 2010;109(6):e26-e50. doi:10.1016/j.tripleo.2010.02.013

Sleep Bruxism, Micro-Arousals, and Autonomic Activity

6. Kato T, Rompré PH, Montplaisir JY, Sessle BJ, Lavigne GJ. Sleep bruxism: an oromotor activity secondary to micro-

arousal. J Dent Res. 2001;80(10):1940-1944. doi:10.1177/00220345010800101501

7. Huynh N, Kato T, Rompré PH, et al. Sleep bruxism is associated to micro-arousals and an increase in cardiac sympathetic activity. J Sleep Res. 2006;15(3):339-346. doi:10.1111/j.1365-2869.2006.00536.x

8. Macaluso GM, Guerra P, Di Giovanni G, Boselli M, Parrino L, Terzano MG. Sleep bruxism is a disorder related to periodic arousals during sleep. J Dent Res. 1998;77(4):565-573. doi:10.1177/00220345980770040901

Tooth Wear, Mechanical Load, and Dental Consequences

9. Manfredini D, Lobbezoo F. Relationship between bruxism and temporomandibular disorders: a systematic review of literature from 1998 to 2008. Oral Surg Oral Med Oral Pathol Oral Radiol Endod. 2010;109(6):e26-e50. doi:10.1016/j.tripleo.2010.02.013

10. Okeson JP. Management of Temporomandibular Disorders and Occlusion. 8th ed. Elsevier; 2019.

Temporomandibular Joint Stress and Imaging Findings

11. Okeson JP. Management of Temporomandibular Disorders and Occlusion. 8th ed. Elsevier; 2019.

12. Tomas X, Pomes J, Berenguer J, et al. MR imaging of temporomandibular joint dysfunction: a pictorial review. Radiographics. 2006;26(3):765-781. doi:10.1148/rg.263055091

Craniofacial Pain, Headache, and Referred Pain

13. Svensson P, Jadidi F, Arima T, et al. Relationships between craniofacial pain and bruxism. J Oral Rehabil.2008;35(7):524-547. doi:10.1111/j.1365-2842.2008.01852.x

Jaw, Neck, and Shoulder Co-Activation (Bracing Patterns)

14. Bansevicius D, Westgaard RH, Jensen C. Mental stress of long duration: EMG activity, perceived tension, fatigue, and pain development in pain-free subjects. Headache. 1997;37(8):499-510.

Habit Science, Automaticity, and Awareness

15. Wood W, Rünger D. Psychology of habit. Annu Rev Psychol. 2016;67:289-314. doi:10.1146/annurev-psych-122414-033417

Biofeedback and Behavioral Interventions for Bruxism

16. Jokubauskas L, Baltrušaitytė A, Pileičikienė G. Oral appliances for managing sleep bruxism and temporomandibular disorders: a scoping review. J Oral Rehabil. 2018;45(1):81-90. doi:10.1111/joor.12558

17. de Albuquerque Vieira R, Oliveira-Souza AIS, Hahn L, Bähr S, Armijo-Olivo S, Ferreira PH. Effectiveness of biofeedback in individuals with awake bruxism compared to other types of treatment: a systematic review. Int J Environ Res Public Health. 2023;20(2):1558. doi:10.3390/ijerph20021558

Chapter 2: Introducing the BRUX Method

From Awareness to Lasting Change

By now, two truths should feel clear. First, your body has been signaling through tension long before pain ever showed up. Second, effort was never the missing ingredient. Awareness was.

So the next question is straightforward: What do you do with what you now notice?

Awareness is a flashlight, not a strategy. It shows you the clench, the breath hold, the bracing. But without a response you can repeat, noticing can turn into irritation. You catch the habit, but you do not yet know how to 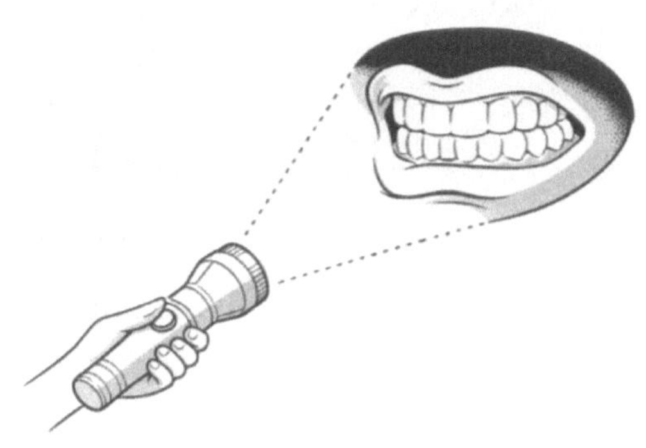 interrupt it in a way that holds under pressure. You are more awake to the pattern, but not yet free of it.

That is where the BRUX Method comes in.

The BRUX Method is a structured path that moves you from unconscious jaw tension to conscious calm in the same order your nervous system learns and updates habits.[1,3] It is not built on willpower, perfection, or constant self-monitoring.

Instead, it gives you a repeatable sequence that makes tension visible, lowers the body's threat response, and then trains a new default through small, consistent resets.

You are not trying to "stop clenching" by force. You are teaching your system a safer option that it can choose automatically.[1,3] Over time, the brain stops treating bracing as necessary, because it has evidence, collected through repetition, that ease works.

The goal is not to become hyper-aware forever. The goal is to make calm the path of least resistance.

What the BRUX Method Is

BRUX is not just an acronym. It is a roadmap that mirrors how habits form and how they change. Each step builds on the last, guiding your nervous system from automatic tension toward automatic ease.

Step	Action	Core Skill
B	Build Awareness	Observation
R	Relax the Response	Regulation
U	Understand the Triggers	Insight
X	eXchange the Pattern	Habit Re-creation

This sequence matters.

Habits are not erased by insight alone.[8,11] They change when awareness, regulation, understanding, and repetition work together.

42

The BRUX Method follows that order deliberately, strengthening a different neural circuit at each stage.

You are not forcing change. You are teaching your body what safety feels like again.

B — Build Awareness

Every transformation begins with noticing.
Before the jaw can relax, tension must become visible.[4,8] This step trains observation without judgment.[4] You learn to recognize the earliest signals of bracing: teeth touching, breath shortening, shoulders lifting, jaw tightening by a few degrees.

This stage engages the brain's sensory and interoceptive systems, especially the insula, which helps translate internal sensations into conscious awareness.[4]

The more you practice noticing, the faster these signals reach consciousness.

Awareness breaks autopilot.[8] It interrupts the silent handoff from stress to muscle contraction. Each moment of noticing loosens the first link in the chain.
You have already begun this step. Every time you ask, "Are my teeth touching?" you are building awareness.

R — Relax the Response

Once tension is visible, the next task is response.
Relaxation here is not collapse or passivity. It is precise regulation. When you separate your teeth, soften your jaw, slow your breath, or

drop your shoulders, you activate the parasympathetic nervous system.[5,6]

This is the system responsible for repair, digestion, and recovery. Each relaxed response teaches your nervous system a new association.[5,9] Awareness no longer signals danger. It signals safety.[5]

Over time, relaxation becomes easier and faster. What starts as a conscious reset becomes a reflexive one.

This is where awareness turns into relief.

U — Understand the Triggers

Tension is never random.[7]

Every clench has context.[7,8] This step helps you decode the conditions that fuel your reflex. Triggers may be emotional, environmental, cognitive, or physiological.[7]

Stress, screens, posture, fatigue, caffeine, rumination, perfectionism.

Understanding does not mean analyzing endlessly. It means recognizing patterns.
When you know your triggers, tension loses its mystery. Anticipation replaces surprise. You stop asking, "Why is this happening?" and start thinking, "I know this moment."

That shift creates choice.

X — eXchange the Pattern

The nervous system does not delete habits. It replaces them.[8,9]

44

This final step is where repetition reshapes your default state. Each time you notice tension and replace it with a calming response, you reinforce a new loop.[8,9] Stress no longer ends in clenching. It ends in regulation.

This is neuroplasticity in action.[8] Repeated calm teaches the brain that rest is safe.[5,9] Over time, the jaw chooses softness automatically.

Neuroplasticity is the brain's remarkable ability to reorganize itself by forming new neural connections throughout life, allowing it to adapt, learn, and recover from injury or disease by changing its structure and function in response to experiences and environment. You are not erasing the old habit. You are upgrading it.

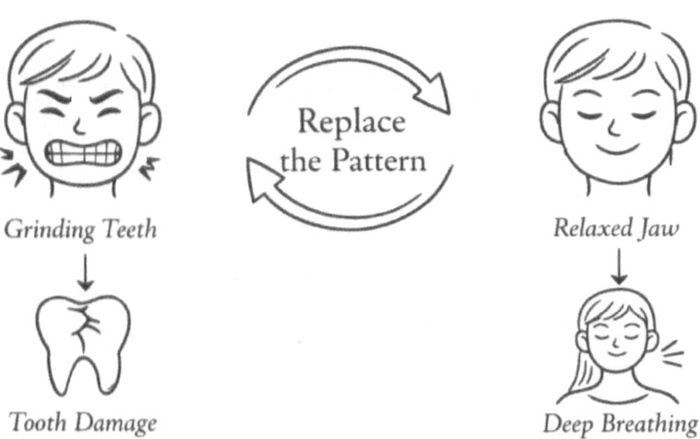

Why You Need a Framework

Without structure, awareness can feel overwhelming.[8,11] You see the problem but do not know what to do next. Should you stretch, breathe, meditate, buy another device, or try harder?

The nervous system does not thrive on guessing. It thrives on sequence.

Frameworks reduce cognitive load.[8] They give the brain predictability, which creates safety. When your system knows what comes next, vigilance decreases. Calm becomes accessible.

Structured habit programs consistently outperform willpower-based approaches because they replace effort with process.[8,11] Each step builds confidence, and confidence reinforces learning.

The BRUX Method turns "trying to relax" into a trainable skill.

Why BRUX Works When Willpower Does Not

Willpower lives in the prefrontal cortex.[10] It fatigues. It drains. It disappears under stress and sleep.[10]

The prefrontal cortex (PFC) is the brain's "executive control center," located at the front of the frontal lobe, responsible for complex functions like planning, decision-making, personality, social behavior, impulse control, and working memory Habits live deeper.[8,10]

The BRUX Method trains the same automatic systems that created the clenching reflex in the first place. Instead of forcing calm, you condition it. Awareness paired with relaxation updates the nervous system's expectations. Over time, a new feedback loop forms:

The calmer you feel, the less you clench. The less you clench, the calmer you feel. That loop sustains itself. Your First BRUX Routine.

You do not need to overhaul your life

You do not need a new schedule, a new personality, or a perfect routine. You need repetition with intention. Small, consistent cues retrain the nervous system faster than big efforts done occasionally.[8,9]

Your goal is not to force relaxation, but to practice returning to neutral often enough that it becomes familiar.

Morning

Do a two-minute relax reset before your day accelerates. Part your teeth and let the tongue rest softly. Slow your breath through the nose and feel the ribs expand. Set a calm baseline before screens, traffic, and decisions invite bracing. Start the day unarmored.

Midday

Complete five brief jaw check-ins during natural anchors. After meals, calls, or meetings, pause for ten seconds. Notice lips, teeth, tongue, and breath. Drop shoulders and soften the eyes. You are not fixing anything, only catching early activation before it escalates into pain later.

Evening

Trace the tightness without judgment. Journal when tension showed up and what preceded it. Identify the pattern, not the villain. Was it rushing, conflict, concentration, dehydration, or posture drift?

This is data collection. Awareness becomes useful when it shows you what consistently pulls you out of neutral.

Bedtime

Do a thirty-second drop right before sleep. Long exhale through the nose or with a soft sigh. Let the jaw hang heavy and the tongue relax. Feel the face soften. This is not a performance. It is a signal to your nervous system that the day is over.

This one-week practice is a minimal protocol designed to build awareness and reduce cumulative tension without requiring major lifestyle change.
In the morning, you establish a calm baseline before stressors arrive. At midday, you interrupt the clench early through brief check-ins linked to existing routines, preventing tension from becoming a sustained load. In the evening, you convert symptoms into information by recording when tension appears and what preceded it, revealing your repeatable triggers. At bedtime, a short drop and long exhale lowers arousal and helps the jaw release before sleep.

Do not aim for perfect stillness or a clench-free week. Aim for noticing sooner, responding gently, and collecting patterns. When regulation becomes rhythmic, the nervous system updates its default, and the jaw loses the job of constant bracing.

What to Expect

Change unfolds in layers

Change rarely arrives as a sudden breakthrough. It unfolds in layers because your nervous system learns in stages.[8]

In week one, you may only notice clenching after it has already happened. That is not failure. That is the first visible sign that awareness is coming online.

In week two, you begin to catch the clench while it is happening. The release comes faster because the habit loop is being interrupted closer to the start. In week three, you start noticing the cue before the clench, such as shallow breathing, narrowed vision, a raised shoulder, or tongue pressure.

This is where prevention begins, because the system is being guided before it escalates. Within a month, many people report fewer headaches, less jaw fatigue, deeper sleep, and a quieter mind. Not because life became easier, but because the body stopped bracing by default and began returning to neutral more often.

Moving Forward

Moving forward requires a shift in meaning. You are not fixing a flaw. You are refining a system that learned to protect you through tension. The BRUX Method is not a demand for control.

It is a practice of cooperation. Small, consistent repetitions teach the nervous system that stillness is safe, and safety is what allows muscle tone to drop. This is why progress is built through simple resets, not heroic effort.

When the jaw softens, the nervous system receives evidence that the threat has passed. When the nervous system calms, breathing deepens, posture stacks more easily, and emotions become less reactive. The work is not dramatic, and it is not fast in the way people expect. It is quiet work, repeated until it becomes automatic.

Over time, the jaw stops volunteering as your stabilizer, and you regain more than comfort. You regain energy, steadier sleep, and a body that feels like an ally again.

Reflection Prompt

Take a moment and write your answer to this question:

When you imagine living without jaw tension, what feels easiest to reclaim right now: sleep, focus, energy, or mood?

Write the first word that comes to you. Do not improve it. Do not negotiate with it. Do not look for the "best" answer. Let the first answer stand, even if it surprises you. Even if it feels too simple. Even if part of you wants to argue with it.

This is not a personality test. It is not a commitment. It is not a diagnosis. It is simply a way to point your attention toward what your system is quietly craving most.

If your answer is sleep, you are probably tired of waking up braced. You may be tired of beginning each day already behind. A jaw that stays active at night steals restoration. It can make your mornings feel like recovery instead of momentum. Reclaiming sleep means reclaiming your baseline.

If your answer is focus, you may be tired of paying for concentration with tension. You may know the pattern of leaning in, holding your breath, narrowing your vision, and clamping down without realizing it.

Reclaiming focus means building a new agreement with effort. You can do deep work without turning your jaw into a brace.

If your answer is energy, your body may be telling you that clenching is not just a jaw event. It is a drain on the whole system. Protective muscle tone costs fuel. It raises your internal workload. Over time it can leave you feeling heavy, depleted, and less resilient. Reclaiming energy means lowering the background burn.

If your answer is mood, your system may be asking for relief from irritability, overwhelm, and the quiet frustration of always feeling on edge.

Chronic tension keeps the nervous system in a higher state of vigilance. When vigilance stays high, emotional bandwidth shrinks. Reclaiming mood means reclaiming emotional spaciousness.

No matter which word you choose, do not treat it as a demand. Treat it as a compass. You are identifying the benefit that matters most to you.

That benefit becomes the reason you practice. It becomes the reason you interrupt the loop. It becomes the reason you return to neutral.

Now read your answer again and write one short sentence that begins with: "I want to reclaim…"
Keep it plain. Keep it honest. For example:

- o   "I want to reclaim sleep so mornings feel easier."
- o   "I want to reclaim focus without bracing."
- o   "I want to reclaim energy so I can be present."
- o   "I want to reclaim mood so my life feels lighter."

51

That image is not just a hope. It is a direction. It gives your nervous system a target that feels meaningful. And when your direction is clear, even small changes become easier to repeat, which is how lasting change is built.

References

Bruxism as a Learned, Nervous-System–Mediated Behavior

1. Lobbezoo F, Ahlberg J, Raphael KG, et al. International consensus on the assessment of bruxism: report of a work in progress. J Oral Rehabil. 2018;45(11):837–844. doi:10.1111/joor.12663

2. Manfredini D, Winocur E, Guarda-Nardini L, Paesani D, Lobbezoo F. Epidemiology of bruxism in adults: a systematic review of the literature. J Orofac Pain. 2013;27(2):99–110.

3. Raphael KG, Santiago V, Lobbezoo F. Is bruxism a disorder or a behavior? Rethinking the international consensus. J Oral Rehabil. 2016;43(10):791–798. doi:10.1111/joor.12413

Awareness, Interoception, and the Insula

4. Craig AD. How do you feel—now? The anterior insula and human awareness. Nat Rev Neurosci. 2009;10(1):59–70. doi:10.1038/nrn2555

Parasympathetic Regulation, Safety, and Relaxation Responses

5. Porges SW. The polyvagal theory: new insights into adaptive reactions of the autonomic nervous system. Cleve Clin J Med. 2009;76(Suppl 2):S86–S90.

6. Lehrer PM, Gevirtz R. Heart rate variability biofeedback: how and why does it work? Front Psychol. 2014;5:756. doi:10.3389/fpsyg.2014.00756

Stress Physiology, Triggers, and Contextual Patterning

7. McEwen BS. Protective and damaging effects of stress mediators. N Engl J Med. 1998;338(3):171–179. doi:10.1056/NEJM199801153380307

Habit Formation, Replacement, and Neuroplasticity

8. Wood W, Rünger D. Psychology of habit. Annu Rev Psychol. 2016;67:289–314. doi:10.1146/annurev-psych-122414-033417

9. Brewer JA. Habit change: a mindfulness-based approach. Curr Opin Psychol. 2019;28:16–20. doi:10.1016/j.copsyc.2018.10.011

Willpower, Prefrontal Cortex Limits, and Stress Load

10. Arnsten AF. Stress signalling pathways that impair prefrontal cortex structure and function. Nat Rev Neurosci.2009;10(6):410–422. doi:10.1038/nrn2648

Frameworks, Sequencing, and Sustainable Behavior Change

11. Duhigg C. The Power of Habit: Why We Do What We Do in Life and Business. New York, NY: Random House; 2012.

Chapter 3: The power of noticing

You have probably brushed your teeth thousands of times. You have looked in mirrors, checked your smile, and taken care of what you can see. You may have invested in whitening, aligners, or a custom night guard.

Those are visible actions for a visible problem. But the habit that often causes the most wear is not visible at all.

Clenching tends to happen in the gaps between moments. It happens while you are writing, driving, reading, listening, waiting, and concentrating. It is quiet. It is automatic. It often hides inside qualities you value, such as focus, discipline, composure, and drive.

That is why bruxism surprises so many capable people. It rarely shows up during failure. It shows up during effort.

The irony is that the same focus that makes you successful can also make you sore. The good news is that once you can see the pattern, you can soften it. Not through force, but through noticing.

Awareness Matters More Than Willpower

Most people try to solve clenching with willpower. They tell themselves, "Stop clenching." They attempt to hold their jaw relaxed all day. They try to catch themselves and force the muscles to loosen. This approach fails for a simple reason.

Willpower is managed by the prefrontal cortex, the part of the brain responsible for conscious decision-making and self-control.[1]

Bruxism, in contrast, is run by automatic systems.[3,5] Habit circuitry in the basal ganglia and arousal systems in the brainstem can trigger jaw muscle activity without conscious permission.[3,4,6]

That is the willpower gap. Willpower is also finite. It drains with use. It weakens under fatigue. It collapses under stress.[1,2]

After a day of making decisions, solving problems, and managing people, the brain's capacity for self-control drops. This is why people often clench more at the end of the day, not less. It is also why sleep bruxism cannot be "willed away." Your conscious control is offline.[1,6]

Awareness is different. Awareness does not require you to overpower the habit. It allows you to catch it early, before it fully activates. It creates a pause between the trigger and the response. In that pause, a small choice becomes possible.

This is the core shift of the *BRUX* Method. You stop trying to fight the clench after it happens. You learn to notice the build-up that comes before it.

Awareness is also renewable. It grows with practice. Over time, noticing becomes faster and more automatic. That is exactly what you want, because bruxism is automatic. Your correction has to become automatic too.

Why You Do Not Notice Clenching in the First Place

The nervous system is built for efficiency. It offloads repetitive actions to deeper brain systems so you can focus on what seems more important.[3,4]

This is why you can drive without remembering every turn. It is why you can type without thinking about each letter. It is also why you can clench your jaw for long stretches without realizing it.

56

When a behavior repeats, the brain stores it as a routine. In many people, clenching becomes a default response to certain states, such as urgency, concentration, frustration, or uncertainty.

The brain files it under "background maintenance" and stops bringing it to conscious attention.

This is not a personal failure. It is how habit circuits work. The problem is that efficiency does not care whether the routine is helpful or harmful. The brain strengthens what is repeated.[3]

Micro-Habits Create Macro-Consequences

Clenching is often not one dramatic event. It is hundreds of small contractions repeated throughout the day.[7,8] A few seconds here. A few minutes there. A long stretch you never noticed.

The jaw muscles are built for bursts, not for sustained guarding. When they contract repeatedly without release, the tissues begin to behave like any overworked system. Muscles fatigue.

Blood flow reduces. Tender points develop. Joints compress. Nerves become more reactive.[7,8]

Pain is not the first stage. Pain is the late stage.[7] This is why early detection changes outcomes. It helps you intervene before the accumulation becomes inflammation.

Why Early Detection Works Better Than Reacting to Pain

Pain is a signal, but it is delayed. By the time you feel a headache or jaw soreness, your nervous system has already run the clenching loop many times.

Your muscles may already be saturated with fatigue. Your joints may already be irritated. Your pain pathways may already be heightened.

Early detection allows you to intervene at the beginning of the sequence.[7,9] It reduces the likelihood of the inflammatory cascade. It protects the joint and periodontal tissues before they become sensitized. It also preserves your executive function.

Pain is cognitively draining. Pain increases stress. Stress increases clenching.[1,7] This is how people get stuck in a loop. Early detection supports calm correction instead of emergency response. It is easier to release a jaw that is tightening than to pry open a jaw that is already braced.

Noticing Without Judgment

The most common mistake in awareness training is turning noticing into criticism. You catch yourself clenching and immediately feel frustrated. You think, "I am doing it again."

You feel disappointed. You feel anxious about the consequences. In that moment, you add stress to the system. Stress is one of the main triggers for bruxism. Judgment becomes fuel.[7]

Noticing without judgment means treating tension as data. It is the difference between being a critic

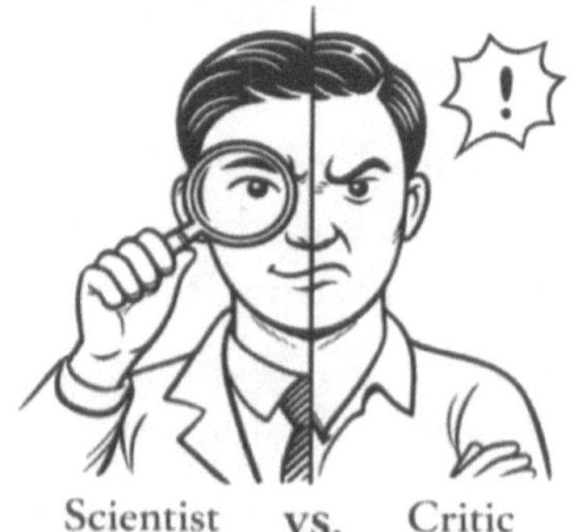

and being a scientist. The critic says, "This is bad. I failed." The scientist says, "There is tension here. That is information."

Neutral noticing keeps the nervous system from escalating. It protects the learning process. The brain changes faster when it feels safe.[10,11]

If noticing triggers self-attack, your nervous system learns that awareness is threatening. If noticing is calm and neutral, your nervous system learns that awareness is safe.

This is not about being gentle for emotional reasons. It is about being effective for biological reasons.[10,11]

From Invisible to Visible

Before you can change a habit, you have to see it. The first step of the BRUX Method is not correction. It is observation. For the next few days, your job is to become a reliable witness to your own pattern.

You are not trying to stop every clench or solve every trigger at once. You are learning when the loop begins and what tends to precede it. Notice the moments your teeth touch, your tongue presses, your breath shortens, or your shoulders rise.

Notice what you were doing and what your mind was carrying. This is not passive. Observation is a form of training because it brings an automatic behavior into conscious range.[3,9,10]

When you can see the loop, you can interrupt it. When you can interrupt it, you can retrain it. The goal is simple: move awareness closer to the start. Once that happens, change is no longer a struggle.

It becomes a sequence.

Pause and Practice

The Micro-Awareness Drill

Do this three times today. Set a timer if needed.

Stop what you are doing for five seconds.

Ask: Are my teeth touching?

If yes, separate them slightly.

Exhale slowly through your nose.

Drop your shoulders one level.

Name the moment without judgment: "Jaw tight. Resetting."

That is one repetition.

You are not trying to be perfect. You are building a skill.

Your Turn

For the next three days, treat your jaw tension like a signal you are learning to read, not a problem you are trying to solve. This is not the phase for fixing.

This is the phase for noticing. The nervous system changes fastest when it feels safe enough to be observed without criticism. When you remove judgment, you reduce the pressure that keeps the body braced. When you remove analysis, you keep the data clean. Your only objective is to collect simple, repeatable information in real time.

Each time you notice tension in your jaw, face, tongue, neck, or temples, write down four items. Keep it brief. One line is enough.

If you do this on your phone, a notes app works well. If you prefer paper, use a small notepad you can grab quickly. What matters is that you capture the moment while it is happening, not later when your brain starts rewriting the story.

Record these four items every time:

Time

Write the exact time or a close estimate. This matters because clenching is often rhythmic. Many people see consistent spikes in the same windows each day, such as mid-morning, late afternoon, or just before bed.

Activity

Note what you were doing in concrete terms. "Email" is better than "work." "Driving" is better than "running errands." If you can be specific, be specific: "writing proposal," "scrolling news," "meeting with client," "cooking dinner," "reading in bed."

Emotion or thought

This is not a deep dive. Choose a simple label that fits the moment. Stress, urgency, perfectionism, annoyance, worry, disappointment, pressure, sadness, concentration, anticipation.

If an emotion is unclear, write the thought instead: "I am behind," "this has to be perfect," "I cannot mess this up," "I do not want to deal with this," "I need to get through this." Do not try to make it sound insightful. Just be honest.

Did you reset? Yes or No?

A reset can be as small as noticing your teeth are touching and returning to a neutral jaw posture. It can be one long exhale. It can be "lips together, teeth apart." You are not grading the quality of the reset. You are simply tracking whether you responded.

That is the entire practice.

Do not analyze yet. Do not look for meaning. Do not debate whether the tension "should" be there. Do not judge yourself for how often you write things down.

If you forget for hours, that is not a failure. That is data too. The goal is not perfect tracking. The goal is growing awareness.

Patterns will appear faster than you expect. You may notice that tension shows up during transitions, during screen work, during decision-making, or when your breathing becomes shallow.

You may see that the same emotions repeat, even when the activities change. You may discover that clenching is not random at all. It is your nervous system applying the same strategy in predictable conditions.

And once you can see the pattern, you can change it. In the next chapter, we will build your Jaw Map. You will learn where tension starts, where it travels, and what it is trying to protect.

With that map, the work becomes less about control and more about skillful adjustment, one small moment at a time.

References

Willpower, Prefrontal Cortex Limits, and Stress Load

1. Arnsten AF. Stress signalling pathways that impair prefrontal cortex structure and function. Nat Rev Neurosci.2009;10(6):410–422. doi:10.1038/nrn2648

2. Baumeister RF, Vohs KD, Tice DM. The strength model of self-control. Curr Dir Psychol Sci. 2007;16(6):351–355. doi:10.1111/j.1467-8721.2007.00534.x

Automaticity, Habit Circuitry, and the Basal Ganglia

3. Wood W, Rünger D. Psychology of habit. Annu Rev Psychol. 2016;67:289–314. doi:10.1146/annurev-psych-122414-033417

4. Graybiel AM. Habits, rituals, and the evaluative brain. Annu Rev Neurosci. 2008;31:359–387. doi:10.1146/annurev.neuro.29.051605.112851

Bruxism as an Automatic Arousal-Linked Behavior

5. Lobbezoo F, Ahlberg J, Raphael KG, et al. International consensus on the assessment of bruxism: report of a work in progress. J Oral Rehabil. 2018;45(11):837–844. doi:10.1111/joor.12663

6. Kato T, Rompré PH, Montplaisir JY, Sessle BJ, Lavigne GJ. Sleep bruxism: an oromotor activity secondary to micro-arousal. J Dent Res. 2001;80(10):1940–1944. doi:10.1177/00220345010800101501

Muscle Overuse, Guarding, and Pain Accumulation

7. McEwen BS. Protective and damaging effects of stress mediators. N Engl J Med. 1998;338(3):171–179. doi:10.1056/NEJM199801153380307

8. Bansevicius D, Westgaard RH, Jensen C. Mental stress of long duration: EMG activity, perceived tension, fatigue, and pain development in pain-free subjects. Headache. 1997;37(8):499–510.

Awareness, Early Detection, and Prevention of Pain Loops

9. Craig AD. How do you feel—now? The anterior insula and human awareness. Nat Rev Neurosci. 2009;10(1):59–70. doi:10.1038/nrn2555

10. Brewer JA. Habit change: a mindfulness-based approach. Curr Opin Psychol. 2019;28:16–20. doi:10.1016/j.copsyc.2018.10.011

Learning Safety, Nonjudgment, and Nervous-System Adaptation

11. Porges SW. The polyvagal theory: new insights into adaptive reactions of the autonomic nervous system. Cleve Clin J Med. 2009;76(Suppl 2):S86–S90.

Chapter 4: Mapping Your Jaw Habit

Up to this point, you have learned to notice tension as it appears. Now the work becomes more precise. Mapping your jaw habit means moving from a vague sense of "I feel stressed" to a clear, objective understanding of where tension lives in your body, how it shows up, and when it tends to escalate.[1,2]

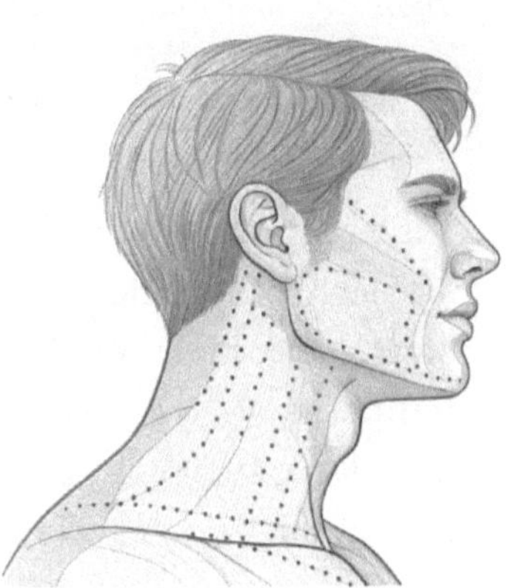

This is not about diagnosis or self-criticism. It is about translation. When tension stays unnamed, it feels overwhelming and uncontrollable. When it is sensed, labeled, and tracked, it becomes data. And data can be worked with.

Mapping is how an unconscious autonomic reflex becomes a manageable pattern.[5,6]

Why Mapping Changes Everything

Most people think of stress as something mental. Jaw clenching proves otherwise. Stress lives in tissue.[3,4] It settles into muscles, joints, breath, posture, and tone.

Your nervous system expresses stress spatially. It chooses places to hold it.[3] For some people, tension begins in the shoulders and climbs upward. For others, it appears first in the jaw or temples. Some people brace silently while sitting still. Others clench hardest during movement or concentration.

Mapping shows you your version of this pattern. Once you know where tension starts and where it travels, you can intervene earlier and more effectively. That is how *BRUX* moves from awareness to skill development.

Step One: Sensing

Building Your Body Radar

Mapping begins with interoception, the ability to sense internal bodily signals.[1,2] This is not mystical. It is trainable.[2]

Interoception is your brain's ability to sense, interpret, and integrate signals from inside your body, giving you awareness of your internal state, like hunger, thirst, heart rate, needing the bathroom, or temperature. It's your "internal sense," linking physical feelings to emotions, such as a racing heart signaling anxiety ("butterflies in your stomach") or a growling stomach signaling hunger.

Three times a day, morning, midday, and evening, perform a brief body scan. It takes less than one minute. Start at the top and move down.

The Jaw
Are your molars touching? Even light contact counts. Muscle activation begins the moment teeth meet. Create a small gap and let the jaw hang.

The Tongue
Is your tongue resting softly on the palate, or pressing hard? Notice suction, tooth contact, or pushing. Let it widen and rest, heavy.

The Face
Notice your brow and eyes. Are they narrowed, squinting, or gripping? Soften the forehead, unclench the eyelids, and widen your peripheral vision.

The Neck and Shoulders
Are your shoulders creeping toward your ears? That is fight-or-

flight bracing. Drop them down and back. Lengthen the neck and exhale slowly.

Do not try to fix anything yet. The goal is sensing, not correcting.[10,11] You are calibrating your internal radar.[1]

Step Two: Labeling

Turning Sensation into Data

Once tension is sensed, it needs a name. Labeling engages the prefrontal cortex, the part of the brain responsible for observation and choice. It transforms sensation into information.[7,8]

Use a simple scale from 0 to 10.

0–2: Resting
Muscles feel soft and pliable. Teeth are apart. Breath is easy.

3–6: Bracing
Muscles feel firm but not painful. Teeth may touch lightly. Effort is present.

7–10: Clenching
Muscles feel hard or knotted. Teeth are clamped. You may notice heat, pulsing, or pressure.

There is no good number or bad number. These are coordinates, not judgments.[7,8]

When you identify a 7 or higher, pause and ask one question:

What was I just doing or thinking?

This question begins to reveal the cue in your habit loop.

Step Three: Tracking

Creating Your Daily Habit Map

To see patterns clearly, you need a short window of structured observation. For three days, keep a simple log. You are not tracking constantly. You are checking in when you notice tension or during your scheduled scans.

Use a table like this:

Time	Primary Location	Tension Grade (0–10)	Activity or Trigger
9:00 AM	Neck and shoulders	5	Reading emails
1:00 PM	Back molars	8	Difficult phone call
5:00 PM	Temples	6	Commuting
10:00 PM	Jaw and tongue	4	Scrolling on phone

This is your tension topography.[5,6]

You are not looking for perfection. You are looking for repetition.[5]

Step Four: Reflection

Where Does Tension Live?

After three days, review your notes.

Most people are surprised by how predictable their patterns are. Look for your hot zones.

Does tension begin in the shoulders and migrate to the jaw?

Does a jaw clench precede temple pressure or headaches?

Does tension spike during mental tasks but fade during movement?

Does it persist even during activities you label as relaxing?

68

Also look for the silent clench.

Some people only notice tension when they stop moving. Others discover that their jaw is braced even while watching television or lying in bed.

These observations are not discouraging. They give you leverage. You cannot interrupt a pattern you do not recognize.

The Escalation Chain

Many people discover that tension follows a pathway.[3,9]

For example:

Shoulders brace.

Neck tightens.

Jaw engages.

Temples ache.

Or:

Jaw clenches.

Tongue presses.

Breath shortens.

Headache follows.

Your escalation chain tells you where to intervene earliest. Early intervention is always easier than late correction.[3,9]

The Red Dot Check-In

A Simple Daily Anchor

To keep mapping active without effort, use a visual cue.[5]

Choose one:

A red sticker on your laptop.

A specific phone wallpaper.

A dot on a notebook or water bottle.

Every time you see it, do three things.

Sense
Where is tension right now?

Label
What number is it?

Reset
Drop the jaw, separate the teeth, exhale slowly, and let the tongue rest softly on the palate.

This takes seconds. It keeps awareness alive.

Mapping Within the BRUX Method

Mapping is the bridge between Build Awareness and Relax the Response.[5,11] You are not yet trying to eliminate tension. You are learning its shape, timing, and logic.

This step prevents guesswork later. Instead of applying relaxation randomly, you will know where and when it matters most. Your jaw habit is not chaotic. It is patterned. And once a pattern is visible, it can be changed. Pause and Practice.

Three-Day Jaw Map

For the next three days, your only job is to collect information. Not perfect information, not dramatic insights, not a full solution. Just clean, simple data that tells the truth about how your nervous system moves through a normal day.

This is the beginning of real change because bruxism thrives in the unseen. Clenching becomes chronic not only because stress exists, but because the body learns to brace automatically and then stops registering that it is doing it.

Awareness reverses that pattern. When you can see the habit clearly, you stop treating it like a mystery, and you stop treating yourself like a problem.

Here is the practice. Keep it intentionally small.

Three times a day, perform a body radar scan. Choose predictable times so it is easy to remember, such as mid-morning, mid-afternoon, and evening. The scan should take about ten seconds. You are not trying to relax yet. You are trying to observe.

Check three areas:

Eyes: Are they tight and narrowed, or soft and wide?
Tongue: Is it pressed, braced, or resting?
Jaw: Are the teeth touching, hovering, or clenched?

Then label what you find using a 0–10 scale. Zero means no tension. Ten means severe tension that feels urgent or painful. Most days will land somewhere in the middle. That is useful. This scale is not a grade. It is a measurement.

Record four things each time:
Time: When did you notice it?
Location: Where are you physically? Desk, car, kitchen, couch.
Grade: What number is the tension right now?
Context: What is happening in your mind and environment? Email, conversation, driving, concentrating, scrolling, planning, rushing.

Finally, use the red dot cue whenever you see it. That cue is not a command to fix your jaw. It is a reminder to notice. When your eyes land on it, treat it like a quiet mirror: "What is my jaw doing right now?"

If you observe tension, simply record it the next time you write your scan. If you want to make a small adjustment, you can, but it is optional. The core assignment is awareness.

That is all.

No fixing. No forcing. No judging.

This matters because judgment is a threat signal, and threat signals increase muscle tone.[3,10] If you turn this exercise into a performance, your nervous system will brace harder. If you keep it neutral, your system will begin to trust the process.[10,11] You will start noticing patterns without needing to chase them.

By the end of three days, you will know more about your nervous system than most people ever learn. You will see when tension rises, what environments trigger it, and what kinds of focus or emotion recruit the jaw. You will also see something else: noticing changes the pattern. The moment you observe tension, you create space. In that space, you gain choice.[1,11]

In the next chapter, you will learn how to relax the response at the exact moment it matters, using your jaw map as your guide.

References

Interoception, Body Awareness, and Sensory Mapping

1. Craig AD. How do you feel—now? The anterior insula and human awareness. Nat Rev Neurosci. 2009;10(1):59–70. doi:10.1038/nrn2555

2. Khalsa SS, Adolphs R, Cameron OG, et al. Interoception and mental health: a roadmap. Biol Psychiatry Cogn Neurosci Neuroimaging. 2018;3(6):501–513. doi:10.1016/j.bpsc.2017.12.004

Stress Expression in Muscles, Posture, and Tissue

3. McEwen BS. Protective and damaging effects of stress mediators. N Engl J Med. 1998;338(3):171–179. doi:10.1056/NEJM199801153380307

4. Bansevicius D, Westgaard RH, Jensen C. Mental stress of long duration: EMG activity, perceived tension, fatigue, and pain development in pain-free subjects. Headache. 1997;37(8):499–510.

Habit Loops, Automaticity, and Pattern Formation

5. Wood W, Rünger D. Psychology of habit. Annu Rev Psychol. 2016;67:289–314. doi:10.1146/annurev-psych-122414-033417

6. Graybiel AM. Habits, rituals, and the evaluative brain. Annu Rev Neurosci. 2008;31:359–387. doi:10.1146/annurev.neuro.29.051605.112851

Labeling, Prefrontal Engagement, and Choice

7. Lieberman MD, Eisenberger NI, Crockett MJ, Tom SM, Pfeifer JH, Way BM. Putting feelings into words: affect labeling disrupts amygdala activity. Psychol Sci. 2007;18(5):421–428. doi:10.1111/j.1467-9280.2007.01916.x

8. Arnsten AF. Stress signalling pathways that impair prefrontal cortex structure and function. Nat Rev Neurosci.2009;10(6):410–422. doi:10.1038/nrn2648

Early Detection, Escalation, and Pain Prevention

9. McEwen BS, Kalia M. The role of corticosteroids and stress in chronic pain conditions. Metabolism.2010;59(Suppl 1):S9–S15. doi:10.1016/j.metabol.2010.07.012

Safety, Nonjudgment, and Learning Conditions

10. Porges SW. The polyvagal theory: new insights into adaptive reactions of the autonomic nervous system. Cleve Clin J Med. 2009;76(Suppl 2):S86–S90.

11. Brewer JA. Habit change: a mindfulness-based approach. Curr Opin Psychol. 2019;28:16–20. doi:10.1016/j.copsyc.2018.10.011

Part II: Relax Retraining the Reflex

Tools to calm the nervous system and reduce the body's default urge to brace, clench and grind.

Meet Evan

Evan is a marketing manager who built his reputation on control. He trusts systems, benchmarks, and precision, and he carries that same performance mindset into his body. When migraines started showing up midafternoon and his jaw began to feel stiff, he treated both as minor operational issues.

He blamed caffeine, screen time, and long Zoom days. He stayed productive, but his baseline kept tightening, and he normalized the discomfort the way high performers often do. When his dentist pointed out flattened enamel and gumline stress, Evan's first reaction was disbelief. He did not identify as someone who grinds his teeth.

The dentist reframed it in a way Evan could understand it was not about grinding, it was about holding. Evan realized his jaw was behaving like a silent stabilizer, bracing under pressure without asking permission. That idea landed hard because it challenged his core belief that he would know if something was happening in his own body.

Evan approached the awareness phase like a project. He tried a phone reminder, but it failed for a predictable reason. His brain filtered it out. The alert became noise because it was not connected to sensation.

That failure taught him the first rule of awareness: you cannot rely on intention alone. You need repeatable check ins tied to real moments, and you need to measure without judgment. So he tracked for a week, not to fix the habit, but to locate it.

By day seven, Evan had something more useful than motivation. He had a trigger map. He could predict when the brace would appear email drafting, metric reviews, high stakes calls, and the quiet, narrow focus that made his breath shallow.

He also knew what softened it: cooking, walking, wider attention, and any task that brought him back into his body. That clarity changed his posture toward the problem. He was no longer waiting to "catch himself" after the headache arrived.

He was ready to retrain the reflex at the front end of the loop, using his known triggers as scheduled practice windows. Instead of fighting clenching with willpower, he could now run a simple repeatable sequence the moment the trigger hit: notice, pause, exhale, return to neutral.

The habit had not vanished, but it was no longer mysterious, and that made change feel both practical and inevitable.

Chapter 5: Relaxed Jaw Reset

Once you can see your jaw habit and map where tension lives, the next step is learning how to reset it in real time.

This chapter introduces the Neutral Jaw Position, the physical baseline your nervous system recognizes as safe. It is not a technique you force. It is a posture you return to, again and again, until your body relearns what rest actually feels like.

The relaxed jaw reset is the heart of the R in BRUX: Relax the Response.

Why the Jaw Needs a Reset

Most people assume the jaw is either clenched or relaxed, tense or loose. In reality, the jaw has a natural resting posture that many adults have simply forgotten. Bruxism does not begin with grinding. It begins with losing this neutral baseline.[1,3] When the jaw no longer knows where "rest" is, it defaults to bracing. Over time, that bracing becomes habitual, then automatic. The reset restores the reference point your nervous system has been missing.[1]

What Neutral Jaw Position Really Is

The Neutral Jaw Position is the physiologically ideal posture for your mouth and jaw when you are not eating or speaking.[1,2] It can be summarized in one phrase:

Lips together, teeth apart, tongue on the roof of the mouth behind your front teeth. This position is not arbitrary. It reflects how the jaw, airway, and nervous system are designed to work together.

To find it just whisper the word "with", your teeth will part and your tongue will settle behind your front teeth on the roof of your mouth.

The Three Pillars of Neutral Position

Teeth Apart

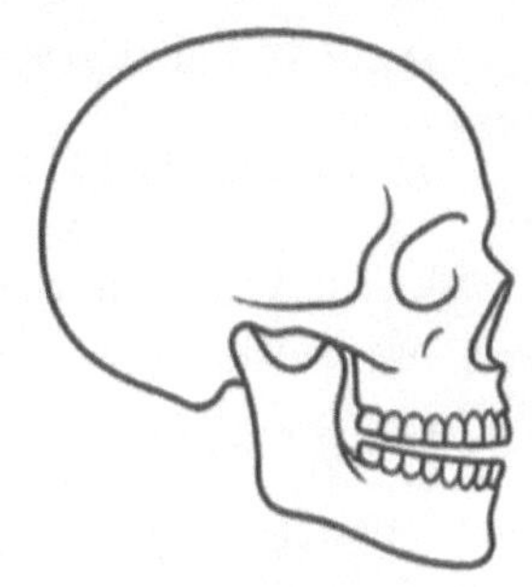

There should be a small gap between your upper and lower teeth, usually about 2–3 millimeters.1 This space is called the freeway space. The moment teeth touch, jaw muscles activate. Separation keeps them lengthened and quiet.

Tongue on the Palate

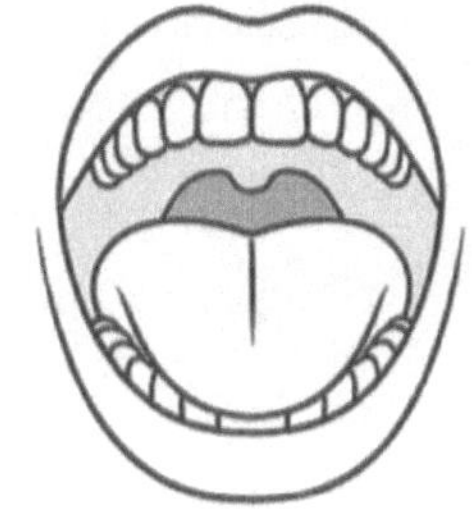

The tip of the tongue rests gently on the ridge just behind the upper front teeth, with the rest of the tongue lightly suctioned to the roof of the mouth. This stabilizes the jaw and physically blocks clenching.

Lips Together

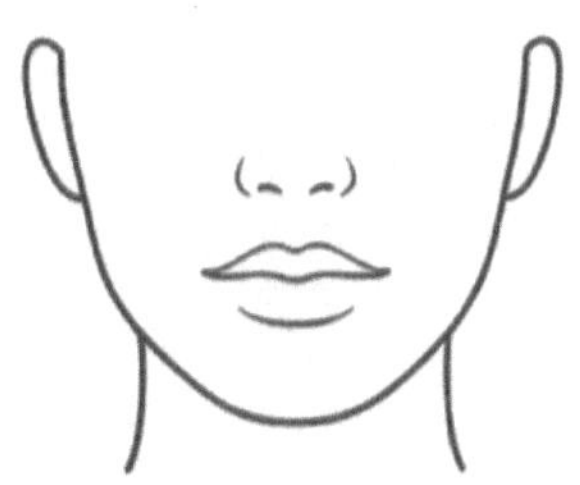

The lips remain lightly sealed without strain. This supports nasal breathing and prevents unnecessary facial tension.

Together, these three elements form a posture that is incompatible with bracing.

Why Neutral Position Changes the Habit Loop

Neutral jaw position works for three powerful reasons.

79

It Physically Prevents Clenching

You cannot clamp your teeth together if your tongue is properly positioned and your teeth are separated.[1,2] The jaw-closing muscles remain in a lengthened state rather than a contracted one. This is mechanical inhibition, not mental effort.

It Signals Safety to the Nervous System

Clenching is part of the fight-or-flight response.[4,5] When you adopt neutral posture, you send a bottom-up signal to the brainstem that the threat has passed.[4]

This shifts your autonomic nervous system
from sympathetic (stress) toward parasympathetic (rest).[4,5] The jaw relaxes not because you told it to, but because the brain no longer feels the need to brace.

The sympathetic and parasympathetic systems are two branches of your automatic nervous system, acting as opposites:

Sympathetic system drives the "fight-or-flight" response for stress/action (faster heart rate, energy mobilization), while the **Parasympathetic system** manages "rest-and-digest" for calm/recovery (slower heart rate, digestion, repair). They constantly balance each other, preparing you for threats (sympathetic) and restoring you afterward (parasympathetic), ensuring long-term health.

Keeping teeth apart reduces constant loading on the temporomandibular joint, allowing irritated tissues to recover.[1] Proper tongue posture also supports the airway, improving breathing efficiency during the day and reducing the likelihood of nighttime micro-arousals that trigger sleep bruxism.[6,7]

Neutral Position vs. the Clench Habit

Feature	Neutral Position	Clenching Habit
Muscle State	Lengthened, relaxed	Contracted, hyperactive
Teeth	2–3 mm apart	Touching or clamped
Tongue	Resting on palate	Pressed against teeth or low
Nervous System	Parasympathetic	Sympathetic

This is not just posture. It is physiology.

Why Posture and Breathing Matter More Than You Think

The jaw does not exist in isolation. It is part of a functional chain that includes the neck, shoulders, chest, diaphragm, and pelvis. Change one part of the chain, and the jaw responds.

The Postural Connection

Forward head posture, often called "tech neck," pulls the jaw backward and downward. [8,9] This stretches the muscles under the chin and forces the masseters to contract just to keep the mouth closed.

Under stress, the body naturally rounds the shoulders and tucks the chin to protect the throat. This defensive posture activates the jaw muscles automatically. Clenching is not the problem. It is the compensation.[8]

Even tension in the lower back or pelvis can travel upward through connective tissue, increasing jaw tone.

The Breathing Connection

Breathing is the fastest way to influence the autonomic nervous system.[10,11]

Shallow chest breathing keeps the body in a sympathetic state. It maintains cortisol release and motor excitation, making clenching feel necessary.

Diaphragmatic breathing stimulates the vagus nerve.[10,11] This tells the brain it is safe to power down. Jaw muscles respond by letting go.

The Vagus nerve is the body's main calming nerve. It connects your brain to your heart, lungs, and digestive system and helps shift you from stress mode into rest mode.

In the BRUX Method, the vagus nerve matters because jaw clenching is often a stress reflex. When your system is keyed up, your jaw braces. When you activate the vagus nerve through slow breathing, long exhales, humming, or gentle relaxation cues, you send your brain a clear message that you are safe.

As that safety signal increases, overall muscle tone drops, the urge to clench decreases, and it becomes easier to keep a neutral jaw position with lips together and teeth apart.

Nasal breathing reinforces neutral jaw posture naturally.[6] Mouth breathing drops the tongue, destabilizes the jaw, and increases clenching risk.

Posture and breath are levers. Use them, and the jaw follows.

Why Forcing Relaxation Backfires

A common mistake that many people make: they notice tension and immediately try to force it away.

This usually makes things worse. Forcing relaxation is still an effort.[5,12] Effort activates the same stress systems that created the clench. Frustration adds a second layer of stress. Muscles respond by guarding harder.

In a chronically braced system, sudden release can feel unsafe. The brain interprets loss of stability as threat and snaps the jaw shut again to protect the joint.

Willpower also fades. Bruxism lives in habit circuits that do not fatigue.[12,13] Suppressing the reflex without retraining it guarantees rebound.

The alternative is gentle awareness paired with physical cues of safety. You are not commanding the jaw to relax. You are showing the nervous system that it can.

Small Adjustments That Create Big Change

The most effective resets are small and physical.[4,10]

Tongue Placement

The tongue on the palate acts like a biological shield. It maintains freeway space and provides constant proprioceptive feedback that the jaw is at rest.

Shoulder Drop

Lowering the shoulders calms the trigeminal-cervical nerve network that links neck tension to jaw tension. When shoulders drop, jaws often follow automatically.

Nasal Breathing with Lip Seal

Lightly closed lips encourage nasal breathing, stimulate vagal tone, and reduce motor drive to the jaw muscles.

Head Alignment

Raising screens to eye level reduces structural pulling on the jaw. Softening your gaze periodically prevents sympathetic overactivation tied to visual strain. None of these require effort. They require placement.

The Relaxed Jaw Reset

This is your core reset. Practice it often.

Let your lips come together softly.

Allow your teeth to separate slightly.

Place the tip of your tongue behind your upper front teeth, resting gently on the palate.

Exhale slowly through your nose, longer than you inhale.

Drop your shoulders a fraction.

That is it.

This position is not something you "hold." It is something you return to.

Integrating the Reset into the BRUX Method

This chapter completes the second step of BRUX: Relax the Response. The goal is not to win a battle against your jaw. The goal is to change what happens after the first sign of tension. Most people wait until pain forces action.

By then, the nervous system is already in protection mode and the jaw is already splinting. The reset gives you a different entry point. You meet tension early, while it is still adjustable, and you respond with regulation instead of force.

This is a meaningful shift in authority. You are no longer reacting to symptoms. You are responding to awareness. That distinction matters because the nervous system learns through timing.

When you reset before escalation, you teach the brain that it does not need to brace to keep you safe. You create a new association: pressure does not

require armor. It requires a small, skillful adjustment.

Each reset reinforces a new loop.

Awareness leads to safety. The moment you notice tension, you interrupt automaticity. You bring the prefrontal cortex back online and you reduce the sense of threat that drives the reflex. Even a brief noticing changes the internal environment. It moves the system out of unconscious bracing and into conscious choice.

Safety leads to release. Release is not something you force. It is something that occurs when the brain believes the environment is stable.[4,11]

A long exhale, a softened tongue, lips together with teeth apart, shoulders lowering, and posture stacking are not "relaxation tricks."

They are safety cues. They communicate to the brainstem that the emergency has passed. When the brain receives that message, it withdraws motor drive from the jaw muscles, and the clench loosens on its own.

Release becomes default. This is the long game. You are not trying to create one perfect moment of relaxation. You are training a new baseline through repetition. Every time you return to neutral, you strengthen the pathway that says neutral is safe.[13]

Over weeks, the old pathway becomes less compelling, and the new one becomes easier to access. Neutral stops feeling like something you must hold. It starts feeling like the place your body naturally returns to.

This is why the reset is best treated as practice, not correction. If you approach it with judgment, you add threat. If you approach it with steadiness, you add safety.

The nervous system does not need scolding. It needs clear, repeated evidence that you can meet pressure without bracing.

In the next chapter, you will learn how to understand the triggers that pull you out of neutral posture in the first place.

Once you can name what disrupts your baseline, you can anticipate tension instead of being surprised by it.

That is when the BRUX Method becomes proactive rather than reactive. You begin designing your day so you do not repeatedly fall into the same patterns.

For now, keep returning to neutral. Not as a performance, but as a homecoming. You are not undoing damage in a single moment. You are teaching your body where home is again, one safe repetition at a time.

References

Neutral Jaw Position, Freeway Space, and Muscle Activity

1. Okeson JP. Management of Temporomandibular Disorders and Occlusion. 8th ed. Elsevier; 2019.

2. Türp JC, Greene CS, Strub JR. Dental occlusion: a critical reflection on past, present and future concepts. J Oral Rehabil. 2008;35(6):446–453. doi:10.1111/j.1365-2842.2008.01819.x

Bruxism, Bracing, and Loss of Resting Baseline

3. Lobbezoo F, Ahlberg J, Raphael KG, et al. International consensus on the assessment of bruxism: report of a work in progress. J Oral Rehabil. 2018;45(11):837–844. doi:10.1111/joor.12663

Autonomic Nervous System, Safety Signaling, and Jaw Tone

4. Porges SW. The polyvagal theory: new insights into adaptive reactions of the autonomic nervous system. Cleve Clin J Med. 2009;76(Suppl 2):S86–S90.

5. McEwen BS. Protective and damaging effects of stress mediators. N Engl J Med. 1998;338(3):171–179. doi:10.1056/NEJM199801153380307

Airway, Tongue Posture, and Breathing

6. Guilleminault C, Huang YS, Monteyrol PJ, Sato R, Quo S. Critical role of myofascial reeducation in pediatric sleep-

disordered breathing. Sleep Med. 2013;14(6):518–525. doi:10.1016/j.sleep.2013.01.016

7. Zaghi S, Holty JE, Certal V, et al. Maxillomandibular advancement for treatment of obstructive sleep apnea: a meta-analysis. JAMA Otolaryngol Head Neck Surg. 2016;142(1):58–66. doi:10.1001/jamaoto.2015.2678

Posture, Cervical Load, and Jaw Muscle Recruitment

8. Fernández-de-Las-Peñas C, Cuadrado ML, Pareja JA. Myofascial trigger points, neck mobility, and forward head posture in episodic tension-type headache. Headache. 2007;47(5):662–672. doi:10.1111/j.1526-4610.2007.00747.x

9. Szeto GPY, Straker L, Raine S. A field comparison of neck and shoulder postures in symptomatic and asymptomatic office workers. Appl Ergon. 2002;33(1):75–84.

Breathing, Vagal Tone, and Muscle Release

10. Lehrer PM, Gevirtz R. Heart rate variability biofeedback: how and why does it work? Front Psychol. 2014;5:756. doi:10.3389/fpsyg.2014.00756

11. Porges SW. Vagal pathways: portals to compassion. In: The Oxford Handbook of Compassion Science. Oxford University Press; 2017.

Habit Suppression vs. Nervous-System Retraining

12. Arnsten AF. Stress signalling pathways that impair prefrontal cortex structure and function. Nat Rev Neurosci.2009;10(6):410–422. doi:10.1038/nrn2648

13. Wood W, Rünger D. Psychology of habit. Annu Rev Psychol. 2016;67:289–314. doi:10.1146/annurev-psych-122414-033417

Chapter 6: Breathing as Feedback

How Your Breath Regulates Muscle Tone, Nervous System State, and Clenching

If awareness is the flashlight of the BRUX Method, breath is the built-in sensor. It tells you what state your nervous system is in before pain appears, before clenching hardens, and often before you realize you are under stress at all.[1,2,5]

Breathing is unique. It is automatic, yet adjustable. It is driven by the brainstem, yet accessible to conscious control.[3] That makes it the most reliable feedback tool you have for detecting and regulating the internal conditions that drive jaw tension.

This chapter will show you how breathing patterns influence muscle activity, why breath holding fuels clenching, and how to use breath as both an early warning system and a reset mechanism within the BRUX Method.

Why Breathing Controls Muscle Tone

Breathing acts like a remote control for muscle activity because it directly influences the Autonomic Nervous System, the system that sets baseline muscle tension throughout your body.[1,2]

It is one of the few internal processes you can change on purpose, and it changes the state of the whole system. When your nervous system perceives threat, urgency, or pressure, it shifts into a sympathetic state. Muscle tone rises across the neck, shoulders, and face.[2,7] Breathing often becomes shallow or held.

In that braced state, the jaw is recruited as a stabilizer. Teeth drift closer together, the tongue presses, and clenching becomes more likely, even if you never consciously choose it.

When your nervous system senses safety, it shifts toward parasympathetic regulation. Breathing slows and deepens. The body stops preparing for impact. Muscle tone naturally drops, and the jaw often softens without effort or willpower. This is why a single long exhale can change your face and shoulders in seconds.[1,5]

Your breathing pattern helps determine which state dominates moment to moment. Short, tight breaths tend to maintain vigilance. Slow nasal breathing and longer exhales tend to support regulation.

In practical terms, breath is a reliable way to lower the background conditions that make clenching feel necessary.

The Sympathetic Spike

Upper Chest Breathing and Clenching

Under stress or deep concentration, breathing often becomes shallow and migrates upward into the chest. You may not notice it happening, but the pattern is common: fewer full exhales, less movement in the ribs, and more holding between breaths.

The body becomes quieter externally, but internally it shifts into a braced, high readiness state. This shift has consequences.

First, shallow chest breathing recruits the accessory muscles of breathing in the neck, upper chest, and shoulders.[3,7] These muscles are meant to assist during short bursts of exertion, not to carry the workload for hours at a desk. When they stay "on," they tighten quickly.

That neck tension feeds into the trigeminal cervical complex, a neural junction in the brainstem region where sensory input from the upper neck and the trigeminal system converge.[9]

When the nervous system receives constant "distress" signals from the cervical spine and neck musculature, it often responds by increasing jaw muscle tone as part of a broader stabilization strategy.

Second, shallow breathing tends to maintain physiological arousal.[2,5] It supports sympathetic dominance and is commonly associated with higher cortisol levels and slower downshifts into parasympathetic regulation. High cortisol keeps motor neurons more excitable.[2] Muscles fire with less provocation and relax more slowly after activation. In practical terms, the jaw becomes primed. Teeth meet sooner, the tongue presses harder, and the clench threshold drops.

In this state, clenching is not a bad habit or a character flaw. It is a predictable reflex produced by an activated nervous system trying to stabilize the body under load.

The Parasympathetic Reset

Diaphragmatic breathing reverses the bracing pattern that shallow, stress-driven breathing creates.[1,5]

When the diaphragm descends on the inhale, the belly and lower ribs expand, and the nervous system receives a clear signal that the body is not preparing for impact.

This movement supports vagal tone by stimulating the vagus nerve, which functions as the primary communication highway of the parasympathetic nervous system.[1,5]

In practical terms, it is one of the most direct ways to tell your system, "Stand down." Once this pathway is engaged, the vagus nerve delivers a message to the brainstem to down-regulate arousal and reduce motor output.

That matters for bruxism because jaw activity is heavily influenced by brainstem-driven muscle tone.[10,11]

As parasympathetic regulation increases, the resting tone of the jaw begins to drop. The masseter and temporalis muscles start to slacken, not because you force them to, but because the nervous system no longer needs them in a guarding role.

Proper diaphragmatic breathing also stabilizes carbon dioxide levels in the blood. This is critical because rapid, shallow breathing, over-breathing, or breath holding can disrupt CO_2 balance and increase neuromuscular irritability.[4]

When CO_2 stays stable, muscles are less likely to feel twitchy, tight, or cramp-prone, and the jaw becomes less reactive to small triggers. This is why breath belongs inside the BRUX Method.

When the breath deepens, the entire system becomes quieter. When the system becomes quieter, the jaw has no reason to stay on alert.

Nasal Breathing and Jaw Stability

How you breathe matters as much as how deeply you breathe, because the route of airflow changes what the jaw and tongue must do to keep the head and airway stable.

Nasal breathing naturally encourages a light lip seal. When the lips close gently, the tongue is more likely to rest against the palate.[1,5] That tongue-to-palate contact acts like an internal support beam.

It helps maintain the neutral jaw position with a small amount of freeway space, and it reduces the need for the chewing muscles to "hold" the mandible in place. In other words, nasal breathing supports the alignment cues that make "lips together, teeth apart" easier to sustain without constant self-monitoring. Mouth breathing tends to reverse this entire sequence. The lips part, the tongue drops toward the floor of the mouth, and the jaw loses that internal scaffolding.

Without the stabilizing effect of the tongue, the nervous system often compensates by recruiting the muscles of mastication and the muscles of the neck to create structural stability.[7,9]

The jaw becomes a brace, not because you are choosing to clench, but because the system is solving a stability problem in the quickest way available. This is why the breathing route is not a preference and not merely a comfort issue. It is a structural input that shapes muscle tone, jaw posture, and nervous system readiness.

When nasal breathing is consistent, the jaw has more support and fewer reasons to tighten. When mouth breathing dominates, the jaw is asked to do extra work, and clenching becomes a predictable outcome.

Why People Hold Their Breath Under Stress

Many people hold their breath during concentration or emotional strain. This pattern is often called **attention-induced apnea**, and it is one of the most reliable "hidden" drivers of jaw bracing because it turns mental effort into whole-body stabilization.[12] It happens for three interlocking reasons:

First, breath holding increases intra-abdominal pressure. That pressure functions like an internal brace, stiffening the trunk to stabilize the spine and keep the head steady during effort.

Once the body enters this stabilization mode, the jaw frequently joins in. The teeth drift toward contact, the masseters pick up tone, and the mandible becomes a convenient anchor point for the head and neck.

You are not choosing to clench. The nervous system is creating rigidity so the eyes and brain can stay locked on the task.

94

Second, the brain often pauses breathing to reduce internal sensory noise. Breathing creates motion, sound, and shifting sensation through the chest, ribs, and abdomen.

During narrow focus, the nervous system may unconsciously "mute" that movement so attention can stay externally directed. This is a modern form of the freeze response: the body goes still to concentrate, and stillness is achieved by bracing.

In that state, jaw tension is not random. It is part of the body's quieting and tightening strategy.

Third, breath holding creates a rebound effect. As carbon dioxide rises, the body eventually forces breathing back online, often as rapid, shallow chest breaths.[3,4]

This sudden shift can spike sympathetic activity, increase overall arousal, and raise motor drive to the jaw. The result is frequently a brief surge of clenching, sometimes followed by a headache or facial fatigue.

What begins as "focus" quietly converts into tension.

Breath as a Built-In Feedback System

Breath is not just a regulator. It is a monitor.[5,14] Your breathing pattern often changes seconds before a clench begins, which makes it one of the earliest warning signals your nervous system provides.

A shift from belly to chest breathing usually signals rising arousal and increased muscle readiness. The body is preparing to "do," not to recover.

A pause or held breath signals bracing, the moment your system chooses stability over fluidity and recruits the jaw as part of that stabilizing strategy.

Even frequent sighing can be informative. It often reflects accumulated stress, nervous system fatigue, or a subtle attempt to discharge tension when the system has been running too hot for too long.

Breath is both a sensor and an actuator, it gives you two advantages. You can listen to it, which means you can detect the earliest move toward clenching before teeth make contact.

You can change it, which means you can intervene without force, equipment, or disruption. A longer exhale, a return to nasal breathing, or a few diaphragmatic cycles can quickly lower arousal and reduce the motor drive that feeds jaw tension.

This is why breath belongs inside the BRUX Method. It converts vague "stress" into measurable data, then turns that data into a practical, repeatable reset.

When you use breathing this way, you are not chasing relaxation. You are responding to the body's first signal that a brace is forming. This two-way loop is the essence of biofeedback.[5]

Using Breath as an Early Warning Signal

Instead of waiting for jaw pain, watch your breath.

If breathing rises into the chest, your system is moving toward sympathetic activation.
If you catch yourself holding your breath, clenching is likely already primed. If your mouth opens to breathe, jaw stability is compromised.

These signals arrive early. Earlier than pain. Earlier than fatigue. That is where intervention is most effective.

BREATH EXERCISES
—— FOR CLENCHING ——

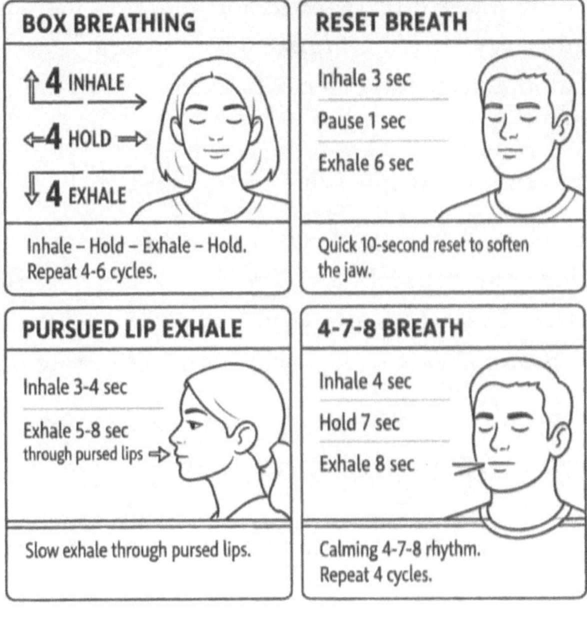

Breathing Practices as Tools

When to Use What

Different situations require different tools.

Box Breathing stabilizes focus under pressure

Box breathing is a simple, structured breathing pattern used to steady the nervous system and reduce arousal.

Inhale through the nose for 4 seconds

Hold for 4 seconds

Exhale slowly for 4 seconds

Hold for 4 seconds

Repeat for 3 to 6 cycles

In the context of clenching, it works by slowing respiration, increasing a sense of control, and nudging the autonomic nervous system away from sympathetic "bracing" and toward calmer regulation, which makes it easier for the jaw to return to a neutral rest position.[5,6]

Reset Breath interrupts acute stress and clenching.

A reset breath is a quick, deliberate breathing pattern you use the moment you notice bracing, teeth contact, or rising jaw tone. Its purpose is to send an immediate "safety" signal to the nervous system so the motor drive to the jaw drops without forcing it.

Reset Breath (10 seconds)

Inhale through the nose for 3 seconds

Keep it quiet and low, let the ribs expand slightly instead of lifting the shoulders.

Soft pause for 1 second. Not a hard hold, just a moment of stillness.

Long exhale for 6 seconds. Exhale through the nose or gently through pursed lips. Make the exhale longer than the inhale.

What you do with your jaw during the exhale? Let the tongue rest heavy, teeth separated, lips together. Think "soften" rather than "open."

Why it works for clenching? A longer exhale shifts the autonomic balance toward parasympathetic regulation, reduces sympathetic bracing, and gives your brain a clean interruption point.[1,5]

In BRUX terms, it turns awareness into a usable response that you can repeat hundreds of times without draining willpower.

Diaphragmatic Breathing lowers baseline tension.

> **Diaphragmatic breathing is a breathing pattern where the diaphragm does most of the work, so the breath expands the lower ribs and abdomen instead of lifting the shoulders and upper chest. In the context of bruxism, it matters because it reduces the "bracing" physiology that drives jaw muscle tone.**

What it looks like

Inhale: Air moves in through the nose and the diaphragm descends. The belly gently rises and the lower ribs widen sideways.

Exhale: The diaphragm relaxes upward and the belly and ribs soften back toward neutral. The shoulders stay quiet.

How it supports a calmer jaw

It decreases reliance on the neck and shoulder accessory breathing muscles, which reduces upper-body tension that can feed into jaw activation. It promotes parasympathetic regulation by creating a slower, steadier respiratory rhythm and a longer exhale, which lowers overall motor "readiness."

99

It helps prevent breath-holding and over-breathing cycles that can spike arousal and increase clenching.

Simple practice (60 seconds)

Sit upright with a soft sternum lift, jaw neutral, lips together.

Place one hand on the upper chest and one on the belly.

Inhale through the nose for 4 seconds, aiming for belly and lower rib expansion.

Exhale for 6 seconds, letting the belly soften and the jaw slacken. Repeat 5 to 6 rounds.

A useful cue is: "Belly and ribs move, shoulders stay quiet."

Pursed Lip Exhale provides immediate physical release.

A pursed-lip exhale is a controlled way of breathing out through lightly puckered lips, as if you are gently blowing through a straw or cooling a hot drink. In the context of bruxism, it functions as a quick "brake" that reduces arousal and helps the jaw drop out of bracing.

How to do it

Inhale slowly through your nose for 3 to 4 seconds.

Purse your lips softly. Do not tighten the mouth or jaw.

Exhale gently through the pursed lips for 5 to 8 seconds, letting the air leave in a steady, quiet stream.

Why it helps

Lengthens the exhale, which shifts the autonomic nervous system toward parasympathetic regulation.

Creates mild resistance that slows airflow and steadies breathing, reducing the tendency to breath-hold during concentration.

Encourages a soft lip seal, which supports neutral jaw posture and makes tooth contact less likely.

Key cues

Lips are "narrow," not clenched.

Jaw stays heavy and loose.

Exhale feels smooth, not forceful.

When to use it

At your desk when you catch "email apnea."

During driving, difficult conversations, or any moment you notice teeth touching.

As a 10-second reset when biofeedback cues you to release.

4-7-8 Breath provides immediate physical release, ideal before sleep.

4-7-8 breathing is a simple paced-breath technique that uses a longer exhale to lower physiological arousal.5 In the context of bruxism, it helps reduce sympathetic drive, which can decrease baseline jaw muscle tone and make nighttime clenching less likely.

How to do it

Sit or lie down comfortably. Let your jaw rest with lips together and teeth slightly apart.

Inhale through the nose for 4 seconds.

Hold the breath gently for 7 seconds (no straining).

Exhale slowly for 8 seconds, ideally through the mouth with a soft, controlled release. Pursed lips can help slow the exhale.

Repeat for 4 cycles to start. If you feel lightheaded, shorten the hold or the exhale and keep the breath smooth.

Why it helps

The extended exhale increases parasympathetic influence, lowering motor "readiness" that feeds clenching.

The hold builds tolerance to rising CO_2, which can reduce the urge to gasp or switch into chest breathing.

The rhythm acts like a pre-sleep downshift, raising the arousal threshold that contributes to micro-arousals.

Best times to use it

Evening wind-down, especially after screens or stressful work.

In bed as a transition into sleep.

After you notice jaw activation and want a fast nervous system reset.

None of these are meditations. They are interventions.

A Daily Breathing Schedule for Bruxism Support

Use breath strategically throughout the day.

Morning

Technique: Diaphragmatic breathing
When: Before work or first emails
Goal: Establish a low-tension baseline

Midday

Technique: Box breathing
When: Deep work, meetings, driving
Goal: Prevent concentration-induced bracing

Trigger Moments

Technique: Reset breath with extended exhale
When: You notice clenching or irritation
Goal: Interrupt the reflex immediately

Evening
Technique: 4-7-8 breathing

When: Fifteen minutes before bed
Goal: Lower accumulated stress and reduce sleep bruxism risk

Integrating Breath into the BRUX Method

Breath belongs at the center of the BRUX Method because it supports change without demanding constant self-control.[13,14] Most approaches to clenching rely on willpower, reminders, and effort. That strategy works until you get busy, tired, distracted, or emotionally loaded. Breath is different. It is a built-in regulator that is always available, always responsive, and always linked to the state of your nervous system. When you learn to work with it, breath becomes the simplest way to lower jaw activity without turning relaxation into another task.

Breathing strengthens every step of BRUX.

Build Awareness:

Breath is a real-time signal you cannot fake. When your breathing becomes shallow, paused, or constrained, it often means your nervous system is shifting into threat mode. The jaw tends to follow. Noticing your breath is often the fastest way to notice your jaw before you feel pain. It gives you an earlier warning than symptoms, and it gives you a clear marker for whether you are bracing or settling.

Relax Intentionally:

The most efficient way to reduce muscle tone is not to force the jaw open. It is to lengthen the exhale. A longer exhale signals safety to the brainstem, lowers arousal, and reduces the motor drive that feeds clenching. This is not a mindset trick. It is physiology. When the exhale leads, the jaw usually follows.

Understand Triggers:

Breath clarifies what is actually happening in the moment. A spike in jaw tension often arrives with a predictable breath pattern: breath holding during concentration, short chest breaths during social stress, or rapid breathing during urgency. When you track breath patterns, you begin to see the true triggers behind the clench. The trigger is rarely "my jaw." The trigger is a state change in your system.[2,13]

eXchange Patterns:

Breath is the bridge from interruption to replacement. You do not just stop clenching. You replace bracing with a new sequence: soft inhale, longer exhale, tongue resting, teeth apart. Breath makes that exchange repeatable. It also makes it practical. You can reset in ten seconds, without leaving your desk, without anyone noticing, and without breaking your workflow.

Most importantly, breath does not require willpower. It responds to safety, not effort. If you try to breathe "perfectly" with intensity, you may recreate the same performance pressure that drives clenching. The goal is not forced breathing. The goal is responsive breathing. When you learn to listen, breath becomes your most reliable guide. It tells you when your jaw is about to brace and shows you how to lead it back to neutral before tension escalates.

In the next chapter, we will build on this foundation and explore how sound, vibration, and stillness can further quiet the stress response and deepen the body's capacity to let go.

References

Autonomic Nervous System, Arousal, and Safety Regulation

1. Porges SW. The polyvagal theory: new insights into adaptive reactions of the autonomic nervous system. Cleve Clin J Med. 2009;76(Suppl 2):S86–S90.

2. McEwen BS. Protective and damaging effects of stress mediators. N Engl J Med. 1998;338(3):171–179. doi:10.1056/NEJM199801153380307

Respiratory Physiology, CO_2 Balance, and Chemoreflex Control

3. Feldman JL, Del Negro CA, Gray PA. Understanding the rhythm of breathing: so near, yet so far. Annu Rev Physiol. 2013;75:423–452. doi:10.1146/annurev-physiol-040510-130049

4. Gardner WN. The pathophysiology of hyperventilation disorders. Chest. 1996;109(2):516–534. doi:10.1378/chest.109.2.516

HRV, Slow Breathing, Vagal Modulation, and Down-Regulation

5. Lehrer PM, Gevirtz R. Heart rate variability biofeedback: how and why does it work? Front Psychol. 2014;5:756. doi:10.3389/fpsyg.2014.00756

6. Shaffer F, Ginsberg JP. An overview of heart rate variability metrics and norms. Front Public Health. 2017;5:258. doi:10.3389/fpubh.2017.00258

Stress Breathing, Accessory Muscles, Neck Load, and Head/Neck Pain Links

7. Bansevicius D, Westgaard RH, Jensen C. Mental stress of long duration: EMG activity, perceived tension, fatigue, and pain development in pain-free subjects. Headache. 1997;37(8):499–510.

8. Fernández-de-Las-Peñas C, Cuadrado ML, Pareja JA. Myofascial trigger points, neck mobility, and forward head posture in episodic tension-type headache. Headache. 2007;47(5):662–672. doi:10.1111/j.1526-4610.2007.00747.x

Trigeminal System, Cervical Inputs, and Convergence Concepts

9. Sessle BJ. Neural mechanisms and pathways in craniofacial pain. Can J Neurol Sci. 1999;26(Suppl 3):S7–S11.

Sleep Bruxism, Micro-Arousals, and Brainstem-Linked Motor Activity

10. Kato T, Rompré PH, Montplaisir JY, Sessle BJ, Lavigne GJ. Sleep bruxism: an oromotor activity secondary to micro-arousal. J Dent Res. 2001;80(10):1940–1944. doi:10.1177/00220345010800101501

11. Lobbezoo F, Ahlberg J, Raphael KG, et al. International consensus on the assessment of bruxism: report of a work in progress. J Oral Rehabil. 2018;45(11):837–844. doi:10.1111/joor.12663

Attention-Induced Apnea, Breath Holding in Cognitive Work, and Performance States

12. Vlemincx E, Vigo D, Vansteenwegen D, Van den Bergh O. Do not worry, be mindful: effects of induced worry and mindfulness on respiratory variability in a nonanxious population. Int J Psychophysiol. 2013;87(2):147–154. doi:10.1016/j.ijpsycho.2012.12.002

Habit Interruption, Biofeedback, and Replacing Automatic Patterns

13. Wood W, Rünger D. Psychology of habit. Annu Rev Psychol. 2016;67:289–314. doi:10.1146/annurev-psych-122414-033417

14. Brewer JA. Habit change: a mindfulness-based approach. Curr Opin Psychol. 2019;28:16–20. doi:10.1016/j.copsyc.2018.10.011

Chapter 7: Softening the Signal

Using stillness, sound, vibration, and gentle sensory input to quiet the stress response and reduce jaw activity

By now, you've learned that bruxism is not just a "jaw problem." It is a nervous system pattern.[1] The jaw is simply where the pattern shows up most reliably. This chapter is about the signal beneath the habit.

Clenching is often the body's attempt to stabilize, contain, or brace. When the nervous system is running "hot," the jaw becomes an easy anchor point. Your job is not to win a fight against the jaw. Your job is to lower the system's need to brace in the first place. That is where stillness, sound, vibration, and gentle sensory input become powerful. They are not therapies you perform perfectly. They are signals of safety that shift the operating system underneath the habit loop.

Within the BRUX Method, this chapter supports:

B — Build Awareness: sensory cues make tension detectable sooner

R — Relax the Response: soothing inputs help the body release without force

U — Understand the Triggers: you learn which inputs downshift your system fastest

X — eXchange the Pattern: you replace bracing with a repeatable "softening" ritual

Why the nervous system responds to sound and vibration biofeedback

Bruxism is often a bottom-up reflex: your body braces before your mind catches up.[1,7,8] In that sequence, willpower arrives late. By the time you think, "I should relax," the jaw motor command is already running. Sound and vibration biofeedback work because they insert a timely

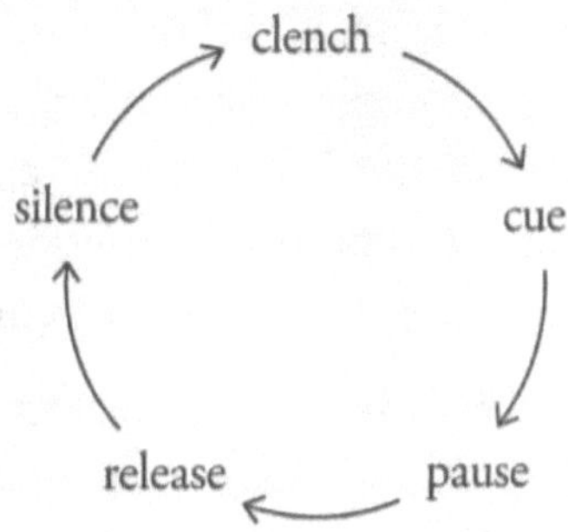

sensory signal into the loop.[2,3] The cue is external, immediate, and difficult to ignore, even when your attention is absorbed by screens, deadlines, or complex problem solving. That signal recruits awareness in real time, which re engages the prefrontal cortex and restores the brain's ability to inhibit the reflex.[4,5,7]

The key is that the cue is neutral. A gentle vibration or tone does not need to startle you to be effective. When the signal is perceived as safe, it avoids triggering more threat physiology.[4,12] Instead, it creates a short window to respond skillfully: exhale, soften the tongue, check freeway space, and release the bracing pattern. Repetition then rewires the system. Each cycle of cue, pause, and reset teaches a new association: effort does not require clenching, and pressure can be met with regulation instead of rigidity. Over time, the baseline muscle tone drops, the triggers lose intensity, and the nervous system becomes faster at choosing neutrality without having to think about it.

1) The orienting reflex: an interruption, not a punishment

When the nervous system receives a sudden, gentle cue, such as a vibration or a soft tone, it triggers an orienting response.[4,5] Your brain automatically pivots attention toward the new input, not because something is wrong, but because novelty signals, "Pay attention, update the map." This is a built-in survival feature, and when the cue is mild, it functions as a clean attention shift rather than a startle. That moment of orientation matters because it creates a brief interruption in the jaw's motor command.[4,7,8] For a second, the system stops running on autopilot. The clench pattern loses momentum, and the brain has a small opening to re-evaluate what the jaw is doing.

Even a short pause can be enough to soften the masseters, drop the tongue out of bracing, and reintroduce a sliver of freeway space between the teeth. This is the critical window. It is not long, but it is reliable, and it is where retraining happens. The cue gives you just enough time to exhale, reset posture, and return to neutral before the contraction escalates into pain or fatigue. With repetition, that interruption becomes faster and more automatic. The nervous system begins to anticipate the quieter outcome and adopts it sooner, often before the clench fully forms.

In BRUX terms, this is the moment where awareness becomes action.

2) Operant conditioning: silence becomes the reward

Your nervous system is wired to seek quiet and avoid irritation. It is constantly scanning for signals that indicate safety, stability, and ease, and it naturally moves away from inputs that feel disruptive. Biofeedback uses this principle in a direct, non-punitive way. It does not rely on motivation, reasoning, or self-control. It simply pairs a behavior with an immediate sensory consequence that the body understands.

Biofeedback uses this principle cleanly:[3,6]

Clench → cue begins

Release → cue stops

The stopping is the reward. The moment the cue turns off, your nervous system experiences relief and registers it as success. This is important because the reward is not abstract, delayed, or dependent on mood.[6] It is instant, predictable, and clearly linked to the exact motor pattern you want to change. You are not trying to remember to relax. You are teaching the body that relaxing restores quiet.

Over time, the "relax" pathway strengthens while the "clench" pathway weakens. The brain does what it always does with repeatable cause and effect: it updates the default. The cue becomes a short interruption, then a quicker release, then less frequent activation. Eventually, your jaw begins to hover in a more neutral position because that state is now associated with comfort and resolution, not effort or vigilance. This is why sensory feedback often outperforms willpower. It trains the habit loop at the level where the habit lives, inside the nervous system's automatic learning circuits, not inside your conscious intentions.[7,8]

3) Proprioceptive retraining: recalibrating what "normal" feels like

Many people with chronic clenching develop an inaccurate internal map of what "rest" feels like.[9,10] Because the jaw has been active so often, the nervous system begins to treat light tooth contact as normal. The masseters stay partially engaged, the tongue may brace unconsciously, and the brain quietly updates its reference point. Over time, true neutrality can feel unfamiliar, or even slightly wrong, simply because it is not the state your system has been practicing. Intermittent cues correct that map by introducing contrast. They deliver an objective, external truth at the exact moment the habit turns on: "This is not neutral."[3,9,10] That message is more useful than willpower because it arrives in real time, before the clench becomes pain, fatigue, or a headache.

The cue does not argue with your body. It informs it. It helps the brain re-calibrate the difference between braced and relaxed, and it

111

interrupts sensory-motor amnesia that otherwise keeps the habit invisible. With repetition, the baseline shifts. Neutral becomes easier to find and easier to maintain. Teeth apart, lips together, tongue resting lightly, breath moving. The goal is not constant self-monitoring. The goal is a more accurate internal map, so your system can return to neutral automatically, without effort, more often throughout the day.

4) Bypassing habituation

Your brain is excellent at filtering out constant stimuli.[11] That is why you can clench for an hour and still feel as if nothing is happening. The nervous system adapts quickly to anything that does not change, especially when your attention is pointed outward at work, screens, or problem solving. Over time, low grade jaw activation becomes background noise, and the brain treats it as normal rather than noteworthy.

Biofeedback works because it is intermittent and contingent. It does not run all the time. It shows up only when the habit shows up. That timing matters because it preserves signal value. The cue is linked to a specific moment of jaw activation, so the brain cannot easily file it away as irrelevant.[3,11]

Instead, it stays salient, which creates a brief window for awareness and a reset. Intermittent cues are also harder to habituate to than steady reminders. They keep the feedback meaningful, reduce sensory "tuning out," and support real retraining rather than temporary compliance.

Softness works better than effort

This is where people get stuck: they notice tension and immediately try to force it away. Forcing often backfires because effort is sympathetic. It adds performance pressure. It creates a second layer

112

of stress ("Why can't I relax?"). The nervous system reads that as threat and tightens again.[12,13]

Softening works because it communicates safety. It lowers the need for bracing instead of demanding release. In practice, "softening the signal" means you choose inputs that naturally reduce arousal, so the jaw doesn't have to be managed with grit.

Four softening tools that quiet jaw activity

1) Stillness: reducing the system's workload

Stillness is not doing nothing. It is reducing sensory demand. When you pause, even for 60–120 seconds, you give the brainstem fewer inputs to process. Arousal drops. Motor drive drops.[12,13] The jaw finds its resting length again.

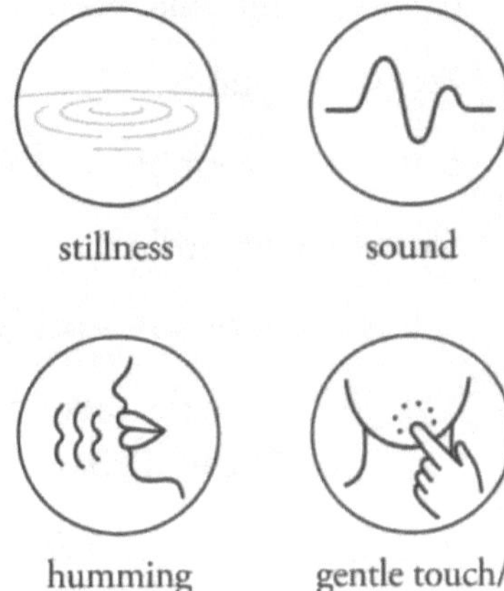

BRUX application:
Use stillness as a bridge between trigger and response. It creates the pause where the habit can be redirected.

Micro-practice: Two-Minute Stillness Reset

Sit upright, feet on the floor.

Let your eyes soften (not a hard stare).

Check your jaw: teeth apart, lips together.

Do nothing else for two minutes. You are not "relaxing." You are reducing demand.

2) *Sound: using rhythm to stabilize the nervous system*

The nervous system entrains to rhythm.[14] That is why certain music calms and certain noise agitates.

When you introduce steady, predictable sound, especially low, even tones, you reduce uncertainty. Less uncertainty means less bracing.[12,14]

BRUX application:
Use sound as a stabilizer during known trigger windows: email, driving, long calls, evening decompression.

Practical options:

Low-volume ambient sound during desk work

Slow, steady music during commuting

White noise or soft background audio during winding down

The goal is not distraction. The goal is reducing the nervous system's "scan for threat" behavior.

3) *Humming: a built-in vagal downshift*

Humming is one of the simplest, most reliable ways to trigger a parasympathetic shift because it automatically slows breathing and lengthens the exhale, which is the body's primary signal of safety. [12,13]

The sound also creates gentle vibration through the throat, soft palate, and facial tissues. That vibration functions as a "safety cue" to the brainstem, helping reduce the motor drive that keeps the jaw muscles braced.

Humming also changes mechanics. To sustain the sound, the lips stay softly closed, the teeth must separate slightly, and airflow has to move steadily. That combination disrupts the clench pattern in real time. Instead of forcing the jaw to relax through effort, humming gives the

114

nervous system an easier instruction: breathe, vibrate, soften. Over repeated practice, that shift becomes a learned shortcut into neutral.

BRUX application:
Use humming as a rapid downshift when you notice bracing or breath holding.

Micro-practice: The 20-Second Hum

Lips closed, teeth apart.

Tongue resting.

Hum softly on a long exhale.

Stop, notice the jaw, return to neutral.

4) Gentle touch, warmth, and vibration: sensory competition

Gentle sensory input can "crowd out" bracing signals because the nervous system can only prioritize so much incoming information at once. When your system is locked in protection mode, it gives outsized attention to threat cues, pain, and internal tension. Adding a neutral, nonthreatening sensation, such as a warm compress, a light touch along the jawline, slow massage over the masseters, or mild vibration, creates competing input that the brain can categorize as safe.[3,12]

That competition reduces urgency. The jaw often softens not because you forced it to relax, but because the nervous system received enough evidence to lower its guard. Warmth adds a second layer of benefit. Heat increases local blood flow, which helps flush metabolic byproducts in overworked muscle tissue and improves tissue pliability.[15] In practical terms, muscles that have been gripping for hours tend to feel less reactive and less "on edge" after even a few minutes of gentle heat. This can interrupt the pain tension loop by lowering sensitivity and making it easier to return to a neutral resting position, especially when paired with slow nasal breathing and a light lip seal.

BRUX application:
Use gentle sensory input after a high-tension block, not as a fix, but as a downshift ritual that teaches the nervous system what safety feels like.

Where ClenchAlert® fits in this practice

ClenchAlert is a training tool: it turns unconscious clenching into awareness reps by providing a gentle vibration cue when bite pressure is detected, prompting a reset to "lips together, teeth apart." In this chapter, ClenchAlert serves a specific role:

It provides an intermittent sensory interrupt (pattern interruption)

It reinforces operant learning: release restores silence

It supports proprioceptive recalibration: neutral becomes familiar

It reduces reliance on willpower by giving you a cue you cannot "forget"

It pairs especially well with softness tools.

The vibration prompts awareness; stillness/sound/humming lower

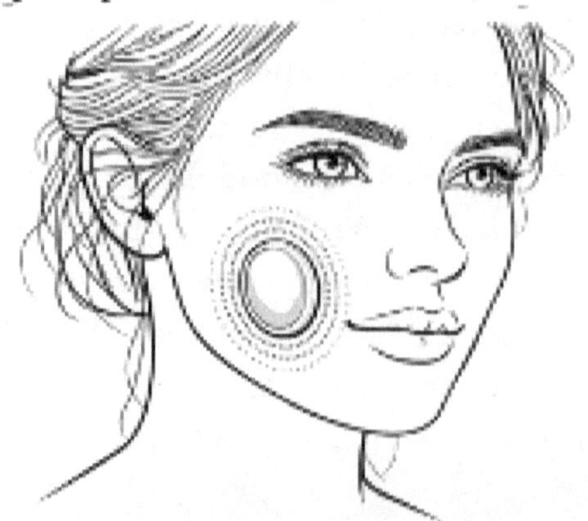

the system's baseline, so the cue happens less often.[2,3,6]

The Softening Stack

A 60-second sequence you can repeat anywhere

This is not a meditation. It is a repeatable pattern exchange. Stillness (10 seconds): stop moving, soften your gaze. Neutral jaw (instant): lips together, teeth apart, tongue resting. Long exhale (20 seconds): slow the out-breath. Optional hum (20 seconds): one soft hum on the exhale. Return (10 seconds): resume task with neutral jaw. Do this once, then continue. Do it again the next time your body signals urgency.

This is how you teach the nervous system: small, consistent demonstrations of safety.[7,12,13]

Softening the Signal: Calm Inputs That Quiet Jaw Drive

The goal is not to become a person who never feels tension. Tension is part of being human. It rises during focus, urgency, uncertainty, conflict, and change. If you live an engaged life, your nervous system will activate. The real goal is to become a person whose nervous system recovers quickly and consistently. Recovery is what protects your jaw, your sleep, and your energy over time.

Jaw clenching is rarely random. In many people, it functions as a protective reflex. When the brain senses pressure, it recruits the jaw as a stabilizer. It braces the head and neck. It organizes effort. It creates a feeling of control in the body, even when the stressor is not physical. The problem is not that your jaw learned this strategy. The problem is that the strategy can become chronic. A reflex that was meant to turn on briefly begins to stay on as a default, and the longer it stays on, the more the nervous system treats it as normal.

117

This chapter is about teaching your body a different pathway. "Softening the signal" means you stop fighting tension with more tension. You stop using force, urgency, and self-criticism to produce relaxation. Instead, you introduce inputs that the nervous system naturally interprets as safe. Stillness, gentle sound, soothing vibration, warmth, slow exhale, and light sensory grounding help the brainstem shift out of threat mode without requiring you to think your way out of it.

These cues quiet the arousal centers that feed jaw activity. They lower the baseline tone that makes clenching feel inevitable. Softening is not passive. It is skillful regulation. It is learning how to change the internal environment, so the jaw does not have to compensate. When the body receives reliable safety cues, it reduces the need for protective bracing. Muscles stop holding their position "just in case." Breath returns to rhythm. The jaw begins to loosen not because you commanded it to, but because the system no longer believes it needs to lock. This is also why awareness matters. You do not need perfect self-control. You need earlier detection and a calmer response. The earlier you notice tension, the smaller the adjustment required.

A gentle cue, including biofeedback, can create that moment of noticing without judgment. From there, you practice a simple reset and move on. Over time, that repetition teaches your nervous system that it can meet pressure and return to neutral. When the system feels safe, the jaw stops volunteering for a job it was never meant to do.

References

Bruxism as a Nervous-System Pattern and Biofeedback Rationale

1. Lobbezoo F, Ahlberg J, Raphael KG, et al. International consensus on the assessment of bruxism: report of a work in progress. J Oral Rehabil. 2018;45(11):837–844. doi:10.1111/joor.12663

2. de Albuquerque Vieira R, Oliveira-Souza AIS, Hahn L, Bähr S, Armijo-Olivo S, Ferreira PH. Effectiveness of biofeedback in individuals with awake bruxism compared to other types of treatment: a systematic review. Int J Environ Res Public Health. 2023;20(2):1558. doi:10.3390/ijerph20021558

3. Schwartz MS, Andrasik F, eds. Biofeedback: A Practitioner's Guide. 4th ed. Guilford Press; 2017.

Orienting Reflex and Attention Re-Engagement

4. Sokolov EN. Perception and the Conditioned Reflex. Pergamon Press; 1963.
5. Näätänen R. The role of attention in auditory information processing as revealed by event-related potentials and other brain measures of cognitive function. Behav Brain Sci. 1990;13(2):201–288.

Operant Conditioning and Contingent Feedback Loops

6. Skinner BF. Science and Human Behavior. Macmillan; 1953.

Habit Circuits, Automaticity, and Pattern Replacement

7. Wood W, Rünger D. Psychology of habit. Annu Rev Psychol. 2016;67:289–314. doi:10.1146/annurev-psych-122414-033417

8. Graybiel AM. Habits, rituals, and the evaluative brain. Annu Rev Neurosci. 2008;31:359–387. doi:10.1146/annurev.neuro.29.051605.112851

Proprioception, Interoception, and Internal State Mapping

9. Proske U, Gandevia SC. The proprioceptive senses: their roles in signaling body shape, body position and movement, and muscle force. Physiol Rev. 2012;92(4):1651–1697. doi:10.1152/physrev.00048.2011

10. Craig AD. How do you feel—now? The anterior insula and human awareness. Nat Rev Neurosci. 2009;10(1):59–70. doi:10.1038/nrn2555

Habituation and Why Intermittent Cues Stay Salient

11. Rankin CH, Abrams T, Barry RJ, et al. Habituation revisited: an updated and revised description of the behavioral characteristics of habituation. Neurobiol Learn Mem. 2009;92(2):135–138. doi:10.1016/j.nlm.2008.09.012

Autonomic Downshift, Vagal Regulation, and Exhale-Led Calming

12. Porges SW. The polyvagal theory: new insights into adaptive reactions of the autonomic nervous system. Cleve Clin J Med. 2009;76(Suppl 2):S86–S90.

13. Lehrer PM, Gevirtz R. Heart rate variability biofeedback:
    how and why does it work? Front Psychol. 2014;5:756.
    doi:10.3389/fpsyg.2014.00756

Rhythm, Sound, and Physiologic Entrainment

14. Thaut MH. Rhythm, Music, and the Brain: Scientific
    Foundations and Clinical Applications. Routledge; 2005.

Superficial Heat, Tissue Comfort, and Muscle Reactivity

15. Nadler SF, Steiner DJ, Erasala GN, Hengehold DA, Abeln
    SB, Weingand KW. Continuous low-level heatwrap therapy
    for treating acute nonspecific low back pain. Arch Phys
    Med Rehabil. 2003;84(3):329–334.

Part III: Understand: Decoding Your Triggers

Go beyond symptoms to understand what fuels tension from within and around you.

Meet Alex.

Alex, a 37-year-old engineer, had lived with jaw clicking and morning tightness for years. It was not constant pain, but it was persistent. His jaw felt stiff when he woke up, and it sometimes clicked when he yawned or chewed. He did what most people do. He asked his dentist, worried something might be structurally wrong. The exam ruled out obvious damage, which was reassuring, but it did not change the daily tension. The pattern remained.

Over time, Alex normalized it. He worked around the discomfort, avoided certain foods on bad days, and stretched his neck during long work blocks. The symptoms became background noise.

The turning point was unexpectedly simple. One night, Alex was reading in bed when his partner looked over and asked, "Why are your teeth touching right now? You're not talking or chewing."

Alex laughed, then paused. He realized he did not know. He was not "clenching" in the dramatic sense. He was just holding contact, lightly but constantly. A low-level bracing pattern he had never noticed. The next morning, he tried a small experiment: lips together, teeth apart. He did not force his jaw open. He simply allowed a natural gap. Within seconds, his face felt lighter. His jaw muscles softened, and his breathing felt easier. A few minutes later, while checking email, his teeth drifted back together again. That showed him the real issue. The problem was not a single stressful moment. It was a default setting that returned during focus and quiet concentration. So he practiced in short, repeatable ways. He stacked quick jaw resets onto routines that already happened: after opening his laptop, after sending a message, after getting into the car. No long sessions. No perfect streak. Just small interruptions of the old pattern.

Within a week, the morning ache was gone. The clicking still appeared occasionally, but the tight baseline had eased. He had not added anything. He had stopped holding. That is the essence of this

123

protocol: replacing chronic contraction with habitual ease by changing the default, one small reset at a time.

Chapter 8: Stress, Screens, and Cognitive Load

Why modern work trains your jaw to brace, and how to uncouple focus from clenching

Most people do not clench because they are fragile. They clench because they are functional. They are managing email, meetings, deadlines, and constant micro-decisions. They are scanning for problems, anticipating requests, and trying to stay composed while moving quickly. The jaw becomes the body's quiet way of stabilizing all that demand.

This chapter names the modern clench triad: mental pressure, screens, and cognitive load. Not as villains, but as predictable inputs that push the nervous system into a threat posture—then recruit the jaw as an anchor.

Within the BRUX Method, this chapter strengthens two core moves:

U — Understand the Triggers: identify the specific kinds of "pressure" that reliably recruit your jaw

X — eXchange the Pattern: replace bracing with automated micro-resets that protect productivity

The Threat–Protection Reflex: why mental pressure tightens the jaw

When your brain perceives a challenge, an urgent deadline, a high-stakes email, a tense conversation, it activates the same survival circuitry used for physical danger. This is not metaphorical. It is a biological reflex.[1,2,3] Your nervous system does not separate "predator" from "pressure." It responds to both with threat physiology.[1,2,3]

1) The amygdala–motor connection

The amygdala functions like an emotional smoke detector. Under mental pressure it signals the hypothalamus, which mobilizes the body for action. One pathway of that mobilization increases drive to motor outputs, including the jaw.[2,3]

The amygdala is a small, almond-shaped pair of structures deep in the brain that acts like an internal threat detector. Its job is to scan for anything that might signal danger, pressure, conflict, or uncertainty and then mobilize the body to respond. In practical terms, when the amygdala decides something matters, it can pull your nervous system toward fight, flight, or freeze by engaging downstream pathways that influence heart rate, breathing, and muscle tone.

The jaw is controlled by the trigeminal motor nucleus, which governs the muscles of mastication. Under pressure, baseline tone increases. The jaw becomes partially contracted even when you are not speaking or eating.[4,5] The trigeminal motor nucleus is a small cluster of nerve-cell bodies in the brainstem (pons) that serves as the main "command center" for the motor branch of the trigeminal nerve (cranial nerve V). Its job is to send signals that activate the muscles that close and position the jaw.

What it controls Most importantly, it drives the muscles of mastication, including:

Masseter (primary clenching power)

Temporalis (jaw elevation and sustained bracing)

Medial pterygoid (jaw elevation and side-to-side control)

Lateral pterygoid (jaw protrusion and jaw positioning)

126

Evolutionarily, this makes sense: a locked, braced jaw helps stabilize the skull and protect the airway during struggle.[2,4] In modern life, that same reflex gets triggered by your inbox.

2) Concentration-induced "apnea of effort"

Deep focus often triggers breath holding or very shallow breathing—an involuntary state sometimes called apnea of effort.[2,6] When breath becomes frozen, the body seeks mechanical stability. The jaw becomes an anchor point.[2,6] Teeth drift together. Muscles hold an isometric contraction that can last minutes at a time, especially during tasks that require narrow attention. If you have ever finished writing something difficult and noticed your jaw aching, you have felt this sequence: **focus → breath freeze → brace → fatigue.**

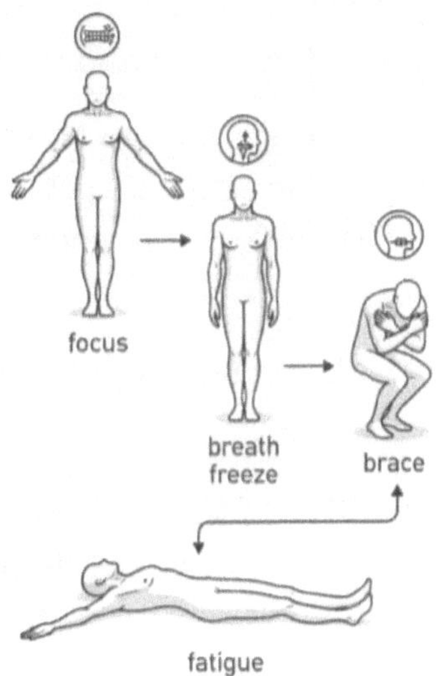

3) Allostatic load and "motor overflow"

When your to-do list exceeds your perceived capacity, your system carries high allostatic load the accumulated wear-and-tear of being "on" for too long.[6,7,10]

Common signs your load is high

Waking unrefreshed even with enough hours in bed

Tension headaches, jaw soreness, neck tightness

Irritability, rumination, "wired but tired" feeling

Shallow breathing, breath holding during focus

Increased sensitivity to noise, light, or minor stressors.

As mental load rises, the prefrontal cortex (the executive brake) fatigues. Inhibition drops. Habit circuits take over. The body "leaks" excess arousal into motor outputs: foot tapping, shoulder bracing, and most commonly, jaw clenching.

Cortisol sustains this state. The longer pressure stays high, the more sensitive your jaw becomes to small triggers. In short: when cognition overwhelms control, the habit loop wins.

Why screens amplify clenching

Screens don't cause bruxism on their own. They create a perfect storm: postural strain and neurological arousal and sustained attention. That combination increases the likelihood that your jaw stays "partially on" all day.[8,11]

1) The visual–motor chain: narrowed focus creates bracing

Intense visual focus, especially on a small target like a phone, pulls the nervous system into a narrow, vigilant state. The visual system "zooms in," attention narrows, and the brain shifts into a readiness posture designed for precision. The eyes concentrate, the face tightens, and the jaw follows, often before you realize it.[8,11]Breathing commonly becomes quieter or briefly held, which further increases baseline muscle tone and makes bracing more likely. This is the same pattern you see in people squinting. It is a tightening cascade that travels from eyes to jaw to neck, then into the shoulders and upper chest. The body is stabilizing the head so the eyes can lock onto a target.

In a modern context, that target might be a spreadsheet, a scrolling feed, or a message thread, but the nervous system treats it like a high stakes task that requires steadiness.

2) "Tech neck" mechanics: forward head posture pulls on the jaw

Most screen use involves forward head posture. When the head drifts forward, the front of neck muscles stretch and tighten, creating a steady mechanical tug that influences mandibular position and resting jaw tone.[12,13]

The hyoid related muscle groups and the tissues under the chin become loaded for long periods, and that load subtly pulls the mandible down and back. To keep the mouth comfortably closed and the skull stable, the clenching muscles, especially the masseter and temporalis, increase their baseline activity. Over hours, that "extra" work can feel like jaw fatigue, temple tension, and a constant low-grade urge to press the teeth together.

This is why desk work can create jaw tension even on calm days. Your jaw is not responding only to mental stress. It is responding to physics. A forward head shifts the center of gravity, compresses the upper cervical region, and asks the jaw and neck to act like a stabilizing brace so your eyes can stay fixed on the screen. The longer you hold that position, the more the nervous system begins to treat bracing as normal.

The jaw braces not only because the mind is stressed, but because the structure is misaligned.

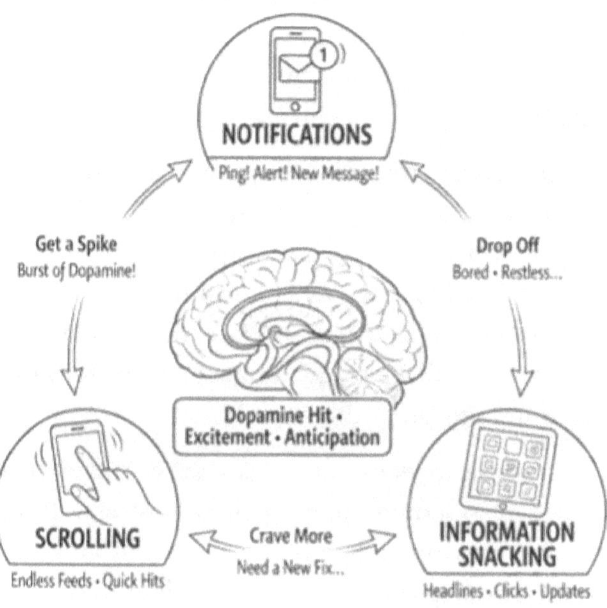

Digital life is built on interruption. Notifications, novelty, scrolling, and information snacking train the nervous system to stay slightly "on," even when nothing is truly urgent. Each ping creates a micro surge of alertness.[8,10]

Each swipe resets your attention. Over hours, that repeated startle and re-orienting pattern keeps the body in a low grade sympathetic stance: shoulders subtly elevated, breath a little higher in the chest, and the jaw quietly recruited as part of the bracing system. Even when the content is neutral or enjoyable, the physiology is the same.

Constant switching forces your brain to repeatedly shift gears between tasks, contexts, and emotional cues.[8,10]

That switching is costly. It consumes executive resources like inhibition, working memory, and self-monitoring. When those systems are fresh, you can notice tension early and make a small correction. When they are depleted, the brain prioritizes speed and efficiency over awareness.

That is where the habit system takes over. Your basal ganglia does not ask permission. It runs familiar patterns that have previously produced a sense of stability, control, or readiness. If clenching has been part of that pattern, it returns automatically, not because you are doing something wrong, but because your brain is conserving energy.

In that state, clenching becomes invisible again. You can be "fine" cognitively while your jaw is working overtime physically. Digital overload does not have to be dramatic to have this effect. It just needs be constant.

4) Blue light and evening load: your body never fully downshifts

Evening screen exposure can interfere with the body's natural transition into rest. As daylight fades, your nervous system is designed to downshift. Heart rate slows, breathing becomes softer, and muscle tone gradually drops. [14,15] This is not a mindset. It is biology. When you add bright screens and constant stimulation to that window, you introduce inputs that tell the brain to stay awake, stay oriented, and stay ready.

Light is one part of the problem. Evening screen light, particularly in the blue spectrum, can blunt the normal rise of melatonin and delay the body's internal "night signal." When that signal is delayed, the parasympathetic shift is delayed.

131

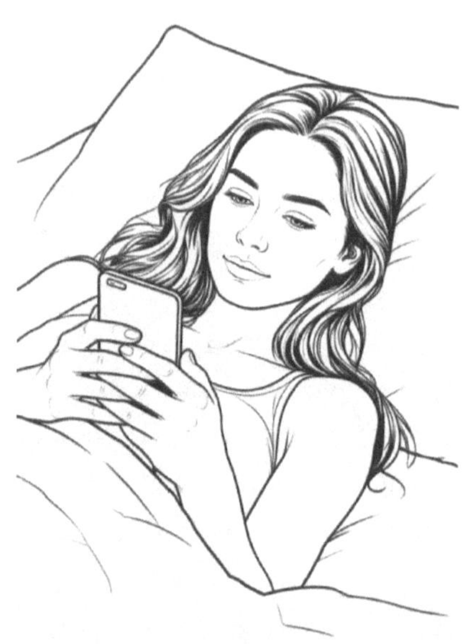

The result is simple and practical: your baseline remains a little too high. You feel tired, but your physiology is still running daytime settings. In that state, sleep onset becomes lighter and more fragile. The jaw, which responds quickly to arousal and bracing, is more likely to stay active during the transition into sleep.

Stimulation is the other part of the problem. Most evening screen use is not passive. It is interactive, unpredictable, and reward based. Notifications, short videos, rapid topic changes, and endless feeds keep your orienting response engaged. Your attention keeps snapping outward, then snapping again. Even if the content is not stressful, the pattern is activating. It trains the nervous system to expect another input. Another update. Another reason to stay slightly on guard.

This matters because nighttime clenching is not primarily a moral or discipline issue. It is often driven by arousal spikes and micro disruptions in sleep. When the system enters the night already primed, those spikes require less provocation. [16,17]

A small sound, a temperature change, a shift in sleep stage, or a brief airway adjustment can trigger a larger motor response. The jaw becomes one of the places that response lands. Sleep onset tension becomes more likely, and the "carryover" into the night becomes harder to avoid. Many people believe they are unwinding while scrolling. Subjectively, it can feel like relief. Objectively, the nervous system may be doing the opposite: maintaining readiness. You are still tracking, evaluating, reacting, and shifting attention. Your breathing may stay shallow. Your face may stay engaged.

Your jaw may stay recruited. The body is not restoring itself. It is staying prepared. A more useful goal is not perfection or total abstinence. The goal is to protect the transition. If you want deeper sleep and a quieter jaw at night, treat the last hour as a boundary that signals safety. Reduce light intensity. Reduce novelty. Reduce rapid switching. Give your nervous system the same message repeatedly: nothing more is required. When that message is consistent, muscle tone drops more easily, sleep becomes less reactive, and the jaw has fewer reasons to stay on duty after dark.

The work–jaw mismatch: why focus often triggers bracing

Focused work triggers jaw bracing because the brain equates high cognitive effort with physical stability. In high-load moments, your body tries to create a rigid platform for the head, eyes, and neck. The jaw is a convenient locking mechanism.

This is why clenching shows up most in:

writing difficult emails

spreadsheet or budget work

conflict conversations

creative output under time pressure

driving in high traffic

gaming or intense visual tasks

You are not clenching because you do not know how to relax. You are clenching because your nervous system interprets focus as threat-adjacent effort.

Turning pressure into awareness without losing productivity

You cannot remove pressure from modern life. The strategy is to use pressure as a cue—then respond with resets that are fast enough to preserve flow. This is how you protect performance while retraining the habit.

Principle 1: Externalize awareness

Constant self-checking destroys flow. You do not want to spend your workday monitoring your jaw. This is why biofeedback tools matter. ClenchAlert® functions as an external mirror: when it vibrates in response to bite pressure, it tells you your mental load has crossed a physical threshold. That vibration buys you a short window, about 10 seconds, to reset before the clench turns into fatigue.[18,19]

You do not have to "try harder." You just have to respond.

Principle 2: Use micro-resets at transition points

The best time to intervene is not when you remember. It is when your day naturally shifts.

Use "seams" you already have:

hitting send

opening a new tab

answering a call

ending a meeting

stopping at a red light

Each seam becomes a training rep.

The Digital Deep-Work Protocol: Keep productivity high while keeping the jaw neutral

Step 1: Set your screen to reduce bracing

Raise your primary screen closer to eye level.

Bring the work closer to you instead of leaning toward it.

Reduce squint triggers (font size, brightness, glare).

Step 2: Choose one awareness anchor

Either wear ClenchAlert® during your first 30–60 minutes of screen work, or

Use a single visual cue (a red dot on your monitor) to prompt a quick check-in.

Step 3: Use the 3-Point Reset when pressure shows up Perform simultaneously:

Tongue Spot (Anchor): tongue tip on the ridge behind the upper front teeth

Freeway Space (Gap): lips together, teeth apart by 2–3 mm (ish)

Exhale Drop (Release): soft nasal inhale; on the exhale, drop shoulders away from ears

This interrupts the bracing reflex mechanically and neurologically.

Step 4: Add one breath-based feedback rule Your breath tells you when you are about to clench.

If you notice breath holding, you reset.

If you notice chest breathing, you reset.

If you notice your lips parting while you work, you reset.

Breath becomes your built-in monitor. You do not need to think about stress. You just need to notice the breathing pattern that precedes bracing.

What to track in your Jaw Habit Map for this chapter

If Chapter 5 helped you map where tension lives, this chapter helps you map what loads it.

For three days, notice:

Which tasks trigger the most vibrations (or the highest tension grade)

What time of day your inhibition drops (often late afternoon)

Which screen behaviors correlate with jaw contact (scrolling, email triage, multitasking)

Whether breath holding shows up before clenching

Your goal is not to remove work. Your goal is to remove the need to brace while working.

The New Agreement with Focus

High performance does not require high tension. That is the new agreement with focus, and it changes the way you approach your day. Most people do not clench because they are careless. They clench because their nervous system learned an association that once felt useful: when something matters, brace.

When the stakes rise, tighten. When the mind concentrates, lock the structure. Over time, that pattern becomes automatic. The jaw steps in as a stabilizer, a silent assistant that tries to help you think, endure, and perform. This chapter is not about blaming stress or demonizing screens. Stress is part of life. Screens are part of modern work. The goal is not to eliminate pressure or retreat from ambition. The goal is to retrain what pressure means inside your body.

Right now, for many high performers, pressure is interpreted as threat. Threat triggers the protection reflex. Protection recruits the jaw. The result is bracing that feels normal until it becomes painful. The work is to build a different association, one that is both realistic and powerful: focus can coexist with neutrality. You can concentrate without clamping your teeth. You can produce excellent work without recruiting your face, neck, and shoulders as extra "support muscles." Effort can be clean. It can be directed into the task rather than leaked into the body as tension.

This is not a motivational idea. It is a training goal for the nervous system. In practice, that new association begins with awareness. You start to notice the specific moments when focus turns into bracing. The first email of the day. The difficult paragraph. The spreadsheet that requires precision. The call you cannot get wrong. Each of these moments becomes a mirror. Not a reason for self-criticism, but a cue to return to your baseline.

Then you replace. Not with force, but with a simple, repeatable reset that teaches safety. Soften the eyes. Let the tongue rest. Exhale slowly. Lift the sternum. Create a few millimeters of space between the teeth. These are small actions, but they send a large message to the brainstem: we are engaged, not endangered. Over time, your system learns that it can stay effective without bracing for impact.

That is the deeper promise: pressure can become a cue for safety, not a trigger for tightening. The moment you feel the urge to clamp down, you treat it as information. Something in your system is loading up. Instead of pushing harder, you respond earlier. You make a skillful adjustment. You protect the body that is carrying your goals. That is the BRUX Method in real life. You keep living your life. You

137

keep working, building, parenting, creating, and performing. You simply stop asking your jaw to pay the price. Focus remains. Output remains. What changes is the internal tone. The work gets done, but the body stays on your side.

References

Stress physiology and threat circuitry (amygdala–hypothalamus; autonomic arousal)

1. Harvard Health Publishing. Understanding the stress response. Harvard Health Publishing. Updated April 3, 2024. Accessed January 8, 2026.

2. Godoy LD, Rossignoli MT, Delfino-Pereira P, Garcia-Cairasco N, de Lima Umeoka EH. A comprehensive overview on stress neurobiology: basic concepts and clinical implications. Front Behav Neurosci. 2018;12:127. doi:10.3389/fnbeh.2018.00127

3. Chu B, Marwaha R. Physiology, Stress Reaction. In: StatPearls. Treasure Island, FL: StatPearls Publishing; 2024. Accessed January 8, 2026.

Trigeminal motor control and jaw musculature (brainstem nucleus; muscles of mastication)

4. Price S, Berrios R. Neuroanatomy, Trigeminal Nucleus. In: StatPearls. Treasure Island, FL: StatPearls Publishing; 2023. Accessed January 8, 2026.

5. Huff T, Mahabadi N, Tadi P. Neuroanatomy, Cranial Nerve 5 (Trigeminal). In: StatPearls. Treasure Island, FL: StatPearls Publishing; 2024. Accessed January 8, 2026.

Allostasis and allostatic load (sustained demand; cumulative "wear and tear")

6. McEwen BS. Stress, adaptation, and disease: allostasis and allostatic load. Ann N Y Acad Sci. 1998;840:33-44.

7. Pfaltz MC, Plichta MM, Blechert J. Allostatic load and allostatic overload. Front Psychiatry. 2023. Accessed January 8, 2026.

Cognitive load, task switching, and habit circuitry (executive depletion; basal ganglia)

8. Monsell S. Task switching. Trends Cogn Sci. 2003;7(3):134-140. doi:10.1016/S1364-6613(03)00028-7

9. Graybiel AM. The basal ganglia and chunking of action repertoires. Neurobiol Learn Mem. 1998;70(1-2):119-136.

10. Seger CA, Spiering BJ. A critical review of habit learning and the basal ganglia. Front Syst Neurosci. 2011;5:66. doi:10.3389/fnsys.2011.00066

Screens, posture, and jaw loading (VDT exposure; forward head posture; masticatory activity)

11. Zaitsu T, et al. Association of visual display terminal time with prevalence of temporomandibular disorder among Japanese workers. [Journal/source as hosted on PMC]. 2022. Accessed January 8, 2026.

12. Minervini G, et al. Correlation between temporomandibular disorders (TMD) and posture: narrative review/overview. [Journal/source as hosted on PMC]. 2023. Accessed January 8, 2026.

13. Xu L, et al. Head and neck posture influences masticatory muscle activity: review/overview. Ann Palliat Med.2021. Accessed January 8, 2026.

Blue light, circadian timing, and evening downshift (melatonin/circadian disruption context)

14. Tosini G, Ferguson I, Tsubota K. Effects of blue light on the circadian system and eye physiology. Mol Vis.2016;22:61-72.

15. Luna-Rangel FA, et al. Efficacy of blue-light blocking glasses on actigraphic sleep and related outcomes. Front Neurol. 2025;PDF. Accessed January 8, 2026.

Sleep arousal physiology and sleep bruxism mechanisms (micro-arousals; sympathetic activity)

16. Huynh N, et al. Sleep bruxism is associated to micro-arousals and an increase in cardiac sympathetic activity. J Sleep Res. 2006. Accessed January 8, 2026.

17. Lavigne GJ, et al. Genesis of sleep bruxism: motor and autonomic-cardiac interactions. Arch Oral Biol. 2007. Accessed January 8, 2026.

Biofeedback and operant learning mechanisms (awake bruxism biofeedback; daytime EMG feedback)

18. Vieira M de A, et al. Effectiveness of biofeedback in individuals with awake bruxism compared to other types of treatment: a systematic review. [Journal/source as hosted on PMC]. 2023. Accessed January 8, 2026.

19. Saito-Murakami K, et al. Daytime masticatory muscle electromyography biofeedback for regulating sleep bruxism (study on daytime clenching control and SB regulation). J Oral Rehabil. 2020. Accessed January 8, 2026.

Chapter 9: Posture, Pressure and the Jaw

How alignment drives muscle tone, and why your jaw often "pays" the price for your desk set up.

If Chapter 8 explained how mental pressure recruits the jaw, this chapter explains how physical alignment keeps the jaw recruited, sometimes all day, even when you do not feel stressed.

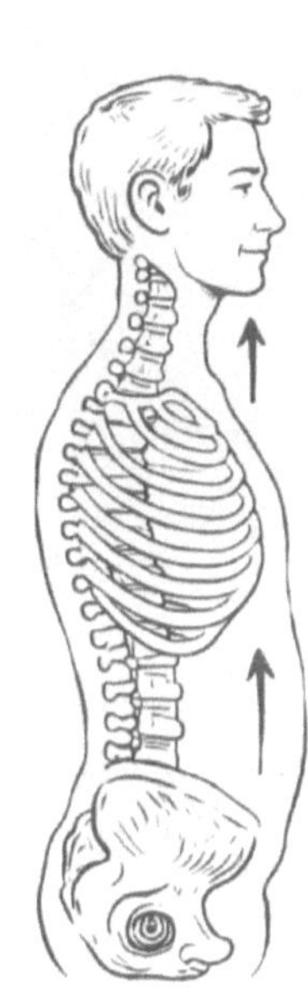

The jaw is not a stand-alone part. It is the top of a stacked system: **pelvis → ribcage → neck → jaw.** When that stack collapses, your nervous system compensates by increasing muscle tone. And because the jaw helps stabilize the head and protect the airway, it is often one of the first places that compensation shows up.[1,2]

Within the BRUX Method, posture work supports two steps:

R — Relax the Response: make relaxation mechanically possible (instead of fighting physics)

X — eXchange the Pattern: replace "bracing posture" with a repeatable, neutral default.

Why posture changes jaw tension (the craniomandibular system)

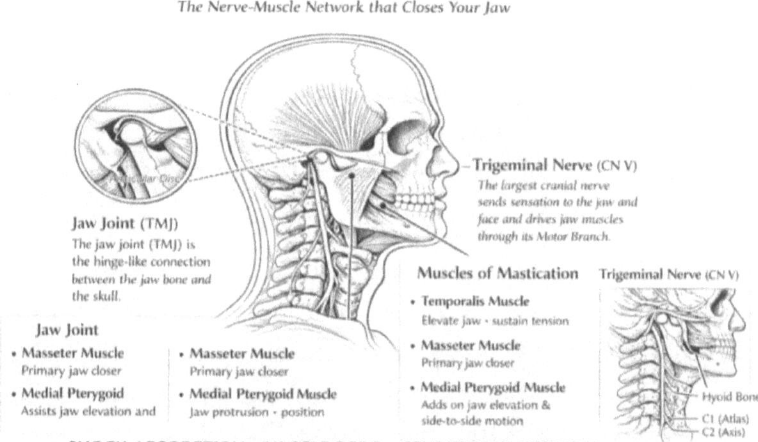

Your head, neck, and jaw operate as one integrated unit called the craniomandibular system. It includes the skull (cranium), lower jaw (mandible), temporomandibular joints (TMJs), the chewing muscles, teeth, ligaments, and key support structures in the upper neck, including the hyoid bone. [1,3]

This network is responsible for everyday functions like chewing, speaking, swallowing, and maintaining a stable airway. Because these parts are mechanically linked, a small shift in head position changes the workload on the muscles that guide and stabilize the jaw.

When posture is efficient, bones and ligaments do most of the structural "holding." Muscles provide small, brief corrections, then return to a low resting tone.[2,3] When posture is inefficient, especially with forward head posture during desk work or scrolling, the system changes.

144

Neck muscles work continuously to keep the head from drifting forward, and that extra demand spreads into the jaw. The masseter and temporalis can become part of the stabilization strategy, increase baseline tone and making clenching more likely.[2,3,8]

When this system stops moving harmoniously, it is often discussed, by your doctor or dentist, as craniomandibular dysfunction (CMD). Common signs include jaw and facial muscle pain, ear symptoms, and tension-type headaches.[1,8]

Forward Head Posture and the Jaw

Forward head posture changes the physics of your body. When the head drifts in front of the shoulders, the neck and jaw must compensate to keep you functional. The result is often a predictable increase in jaw muscle tone that feels like "stress," even when the primary driver is structural.

The Mechanical Tug: Neck Muscles Pull the Mandible

Forward head posture, often called tech neck, shifts the head away from its center of gravity. That single shift forces the body to create stability somewhere else.

One of the first places this shows up is the front of the neck. The suprahyoid and infrahyoid muscles, along with other anterior neck tissues, become lengthened and loaded as they work to support the head and manage airway and swallowing mechanics.

Over time, lengthened does not mean relaxed. It often means tight, over-recruited, and reactive.[3,5] As these tissues tighten, they create a subtle but persistent downward and backward drag on the mandible.

145

This matters because the jaw is not designed to "hang" under load for hours.

The nervous system tends to protect closure and stability, especially when posture creates the sensation that the head and neck are less supported. To prevent the mouth from drifting open or the jaw from feeling unstable, the masseter and temporalis increase baseline contraction.

This is not necessarily a dramatic clench. It is often low-grade, sustained contact or near-contact that runs in the background.[1,3]

The practical consequence is important. Many people interpret the tension as psychological stress when it is actually a mechanical compensation.[2,8] In other words, sometimes you are not clenching because you are stressed.

You are clenching because your posture has created a constant drag that your jaw muscles are trying to overcome, minute after minute.

The Neurological Link: The Trigeminal-Cervical Complex

The jaw and upper neck share more than proximity. They share neurological infrastructure. Sensory input from the trigeminal system (jaw, face, TMJ) and from the upper cervical nerves (upper neck joints and tissues) converges in a brainstem relay often described as the trigeminal-cervical complex or trigeminal-cervical nucleus.[9,10]

This convergence is a key reason neck strain and jaw tension so often travel together, and why jaw symptoms can appear without an obvious "jaw cause."

The Trigeminal-Cervical Complex

The Linked Relay for Jaw and Neck Tension

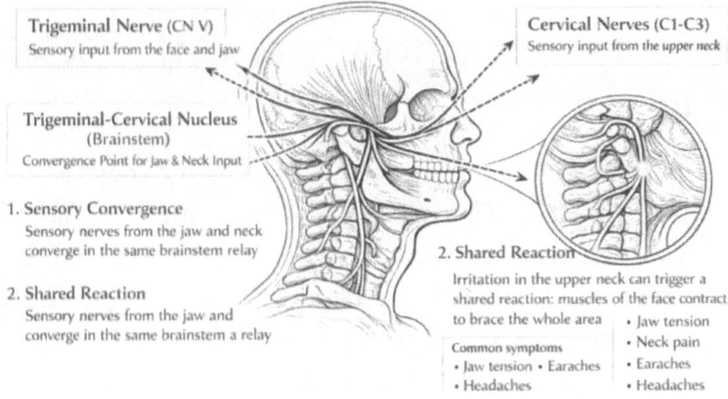

Neck strain and jaw clenching often travel together.

Forward head posture increases compressive load and irritability in the upper cervical region. The joints at the top of the neck and the surrounding soft tissues are asked to stabilize the head in an inefficient position.

That produces a steady stream of sensory input, often interpreted by the nervous system as mechanical threat, instability, or effort. [4,6,10]

Because this sensory traffic feeds into the same relay network involved in jaw control, the brain can respond with a protective strategy that includes increased jaw muscle tone. This protective response is rarely conscious.

The system is not "deciding" to clench. It is tightening to create a brace, an anchor point that helps the head and neck feel more secure. In that sense, jaw tension is sometimes a stabilization reflex, not a behavioral choice. It can be triggered by posture, sustained attention, or neck discomfort, even when mood is calm. [6,7]

This also explains why jaw pain can feel mysterious. The jaw may be the site of symptoms, but the driver may be cervical overload. When the relay station is repeatedly fed distress signals from the neck, the jaw often becomes the downstream muscle group that takes the hit.

Joint Consequences: The TMJ Tracks Under a Different Load

Forward head posture does not only change muscle tone. It changes joint mechanics. When the head is positioned forward, the mandible is subtly pulled out of its ideal relationship with the temporomandibular joint. [1,3] The jaw may sit slightly differently in the joint space, and the muscles guiding movement may pull on the condyle and disc under altered vectors.

None of this requires a dramatic misalignment to matter. Small changes repeated thousands of times per day are enough to shift load.

When you open and close your mouth while the head is forward, the TMJ often has to "track" under compromised mechanics. The jaw is moving, but it is moving while the cervical spine is compressed, the ribcage may be collapsed, and the anterior neck tissues are tense.

The result can be a change in the pathway the joint takes during opening, chewing, or speaking. Over time, that altered pathway can contribute to clicking, popping, or irritation in the joint and surrounding tissues.

It is critical to interpret these signs accurately. Clicking is not always damage, and it does not automatically mean the joint is degenerating. Often it is evidence that the joint is being asked to function under an altered load. The jaw is doing its job, but it is doing it from a position that makes the work harder.[1,8]

When alignment improves, the jaw's resting position stabilizes, the muscle vectors normalize, and the TMJ often tracks with less friction and less protective bracing. In many cases, the joint does not need a complex fix. It needs a better operating environment.

148

Desk work combines four inputs that bias your system toward bracing:

Forward head and rounded shoulders: mechanical tug on the jaw

Shallow breathing / "email apnea": the body becomes static and locks for stability

High cognitive load: motor overflow increases jaw drive

Narrow visual focus: focal bracing tightens face and jaw

This is why people often feel worst at:

mid-morning email triage

afternoon spreadsheets and deadlines

long meetings

driving home in traffic after a screen-heavy day

The jaw is simply the visible endpoint of an overloaded posture and nervous system equation.[2,3,8]

Alignment is a master switch for muscle tone

Your nervous system is constantly asking one question: "How do I keep this body upright with the least energy?" When your "blocks" are stacked (pelvis, ribcage, head), the answer is: very little muscle tone.

When the blocks are shifted (slumped pelvis, collapsed chest, forward head), the answer is: recruit muscles continuously.[5,6]

That continuous recruitment becomes your new baseline, your nervous system's "set point." And once that set point is high, the jaw is far more likely to stay partially activated even outside obvious stress.

The three posture changes that reduce jaw tension fastest

These are not "perfect posture" rules. They are high-return adjustments, small shifts that unload the jaw without making you rigid.

1) Sternum Lift (foundation without strain)

Instead of pulling shoulders back, lightly lift your breastbone up and forward (as if a string is attached).

Opens the chest

Lets shoulders drop

Gives the neck a stable base

When the chest lifts, the head often comes back without force, and the jaw loses the need to brace.[3,8,10]

2) Axial Extension (decompress the upper neck)

Imagine a string lifting the crown of your head. Then make a tiny "chin glide" straight back (not down). Think: lengthen the back of the neck. This reduces the compressive input that drives the trigeminal-cervical bracing reflex and often creates an immediate jaw "drop."

3) Pelvic "Sit Bone" reset (stack from the bottom)

If you sit on your tailbone, your spine collapses. Shift onto your sit bones and let your knees be slightly lower than hips when possible. A neutral pelvis restores the spine's natural curves, which supports the head without muscular gripping. When the stack improves, the jaw can stop acting like a support beam.

The Posture-to-Jaw Exchange: a BRUX-friendly micro-routine

Use this as your Chapter 9 "X" practice, your replacement pattern during desk work.

Whenever you hit a trigger (or ClenchAlert® vibrates), do this in 10 seconds:

Sternum Lift: gentle up-and-forward

Axial Extension: crown up, chin glides back slightly

Freeway Space and Tongue Spot: lips together, teeth apart 2–3 mm, tongue on the spot.

Soft nasal exhale: let shoulders drop as you breathe out

You are not "trying to relax." You are changing the geometry, so relaxation becomes the default.

The Ear-over-Shoulder check: your simplest diagnostic

Several times per day, ask one objective question:

Are my ears stacked over my shoulders?

If not, you have found a likely driver of jaw tone.

Do not correct aggressively. Simply return toward "stacked," then re-check your neutral jaw position.

Most people are surprised by what happens next: as the head comes back, the urge to clench decreases because the tug-of-war ends.[2,3]

Closing: Stop Asking Your Jaw to Solve a Posture Problem

If you only treat the jaw but leave the head forward and the ribcage collapsed, you will keep fighting physics. The craniomandibular system does not operate in isolation. The jaw responds to what the neck, shoulders, and airway are doing all day.

When the head drifts in front of the shoulders and the chest caves inward, the body has to create stability somewhere. For many people, the jaw becomes that stabilizer.

It braces to hold the skull steady. It tightens to compensate for shallow breathing. It clamps to create a sense of control in a structure that feels off balance.

That is why posture work is not optional and it is not "extra." It is foundational support for the BRUX Method because it changes the mechanical conditions that make clenching feel necessary. If you want lasting relief, you need to give the jaw a reason to stand down.[1,2] You do that by restoring stack, space, and alignment so the nervous system can stop recruiting the jaw as a load-bearing muscle.

This is how posture supports each step of BRUX.

Build Awareness means you notice where you brace. Not just in the jaw, but in the whole system. You notice the head creeping forward, the shoulders rounding, and the ribs collapsing as you focus on screens or power through a task.

The win is not perfect posture. The win is noticing the pattern early, before the jaw is forced to take over.

Relax Intentionally means you unload the structure so the jaw can release. When you lift the sternum, lengthen the back of the neck, and let the head return over the shoulders, you remove the tug-of-war that pulls on the mandible.

152

Relaxation becomes less of a command and more of a consequence. The jaw is not being forced to fight gravity.

Understand Triggers means you identify desk posture as a primary driver. Clenching does not come from stress alone. It often comes from the combination of stress plus a position that requires bracing. Email apnea, narrowed vision, and forward head posture create the conditions for protective tension. When you recognize that, you stop blaming yourself and start improving the setup.

Exchange Patterns means you replace bracing posture with stacked posture plus a neutral jaw. You build a repeatable reset: ears over shoulders, sternum lifted, pelvis grounded, lips together, teeth apart. That is the new default. Not rigid, not military, just structurally efficient.

Your jaw is not stubborn. It is adaptive. It is responding to the demands you place on your body every hour. When alignment improves, the nervous system no longer needs the jaw to act like a stabilizer. Quiet becomes easier to maintain because the system finally makes sense to the brain.

References

Craniomandibular system and jaw biomechanics

Supports: jaw–head–neck integration, load sharing, muscle tone regulation

1. Okeson JP. Management of Temporomandibular Disorders and Occlusion. 8th ed. St Louis, MO: Elsevier; 2020.

2. Lavigne GJ, Sessle BJ. The neurobiology of orofacial pain and motor control. J Dent Res. 2016;95(10):1107-1116. doi:10.1177/0022034516648264

Posture and temporomandibular function (associative, non-diagnostic)

Supports: posture influencing jaw muscle activity and symptom expression

3. Minervini G, et al. Correlation between temporomandibular disorders and posture: a narrative review. Healthcare (Basel). 2023;11(3):349. doi:10.3390/healthcare11030349

4. Kraus S. Temporomandibular disorders, head posture, and cervical spine. Dent Clin North Am. 2007;51(1):161-177.

Forward head posture and masticatory muscle activity

Supports: mechanical loading, increased baseline tone, stabilization strategies

5. Xu L, et al. Influence of head and neck posture on masticatory muscle activity: a systematic review. Ann Palliat Med. 2021;10(5):5462-5473. doi:10.21037/apm-20-2381

Cervical spine biomechanics and mechanical load

Supports: neck compression, structural strain, compensatory muscle recruitment

6. Bogduk N. The anatomy and pathophysiology of neck pain. Phys Med Rehabil Clin N Am. 2011;22(3):367-382. doi:10.1016/j.pmr.2011.03.008

Trigeminal–cervical convergence and shared neural pathways

Supports: neck–jaw symptom crossover, shared brainstem relay

7. Fernández-de-Las-Peñas C, Cuadrado ML, Arendt-Nielsen L, Pareja JA. Referred pain from the cervical spine to the temporomandibular region. J Headache Pain. 2007;8(5):341-346. doi:10.1007/s10194-007-0419-5

8. Fernández-de-Las-Peñas C, et al. Trigeminal–cervical convergence and headache mechanisms. Curr Pain Headache Rep. 2010;14(5):404-410. doi:10.1007/s11916-010-0134-8

Neck disability and jaw symptom association

Supports: co-occurrence of cervical strain and jaw dysfunction

9. De Wijer A, et al. Temporomandibular and cervical spine disorders: self-reported signs and symptoms. Spine (Phila Pa 1976). 1996;21(14):1638-1646.

10. Armijo-Olivo S, et al. The association between neck disability and jaw dysfunction. J Oral Rehabil.2011;38(9):670-679. doi:10.1111/j.1365-2842.2011.02206.x

Chapter 10: Sleep, Light, and Sleep Clenching

Sleep jaw activity follows a different set of rules than daytime clenching, and understanding those rules is essential if you want realistic, lasting improvement. During the day, jaw tension often shows up as a habit you can catch, interrupt, and gently unwind. Awareness is available. Choice is available. You can feel the clench, soften the jaw, adjust your posture, or take a breath.

During sleep, those tools disappear. The parts of the brain responsible for conscious monitoring, self-correction, and inhibition are largely offline. What remains in charge is the brainstem and habit circuitry that governs survival functions.[1,2]

This is why sleep clenching feels mysterious and stubborn. The jaw is no longer responding to thoughts or intentions. It is responding to arousal, instability, and accumulated load. From a nervous system perspective, sleep is not a uniform state of rest.

It is a dynamic process that includes brief surges of alertness known as micro-arousals. These occur naturally as the brain shifts between sleep stages, responds to breathing changes, or processes internal stress signals.[3,5]

When overall arousal is high, these micro-arousals become more frequent and more intense. Each surge increases muscle tone throughout the body. The jaw, as a powerful stabilizer of the head and airway, often joins the response.[4,5]

This means sleep clenching is rarely random. It is usually the body's attempt to manage something. That something may be airway instability, nervous system vigilance carried over from the day, unresolved emotional load, pain, or chemical factors like cortisol, caffeine, or dehydration.

The jaw is not misbehaving. It is responding exactly as it was trained to respond under pressure. The BRUX Method approaches sleep clenching with this reality in mind. Rather than trying to control what cannot be consciously controlled, it focuses on two practical goals.[3,6]

The first is reducing the load that carries into sleep. A calmer day-to-sleep transition lowers baseline arousal so that micro-arousals are less likely to trigger strong motor responses. This includes managing evening light exposure, reducing late stimulation, supporting hydration and mineral balance, and giving the nervous system clear signals that effort is finished and rest is safe.

What you do in the last two hours of the day matters far more than what you think while asleep.

The second goal is protection during the hours when awareness is unavailable. Because sleep clenching cannot be reliably interrupted in real time, protecting the teeth and jaw structures is essential.

This is not a failure of training.[10] It is a practical acknowledgment of physiology. Protection reduces damage while the nervous system continues to recalibrate over time. Seen through this lens, sleep clenching becomes less frustrating.

You stop asking the jaw to behave differently while asleep and start supporting the system that governs it. You reduce triggers where you can, you lower overall load, and you protect the structures that absorb force when awareness is offline.[1,2,5]

Progress here is measured quietly. Fewer morning headaches. Less jaw fatigue on waking. A softer face. Deeper, more restorative sleep. These changes do not come from willpower. They come from working with the nervous system as it is, not as we wish it to be.

Within the BRUX Method, sleep care is not about perfect stillness. It is about creating conditions where the jaw has fewer reasons to fire and fewer consequences when it does.

Why clenching often worsens during sleep

1) Your conscious "brake" goes offline

During sleep, the brain changes how it allocates control. The prefrontal cortex, which manages executive function, inhibition, and deliberate self-correction, significantly reduces its activity.

This is the same part of the brain that allows you to notice tension during the day and consciously think, "My teeth are touching. I should let my jaw relax." In sleep, that internal voice is simply not available.

With the conscious brake disengaged, jaw activity is governed almost entirely by subcortical systems. These include the basal ganglia, which store and run learned habits, and the brainstem arousal centers, which respond automatically to perceived threat, instability, or physiological need.

These systems are fast, efficient, and protective, but they do not evaluate nuance. They act first and ask no questions.

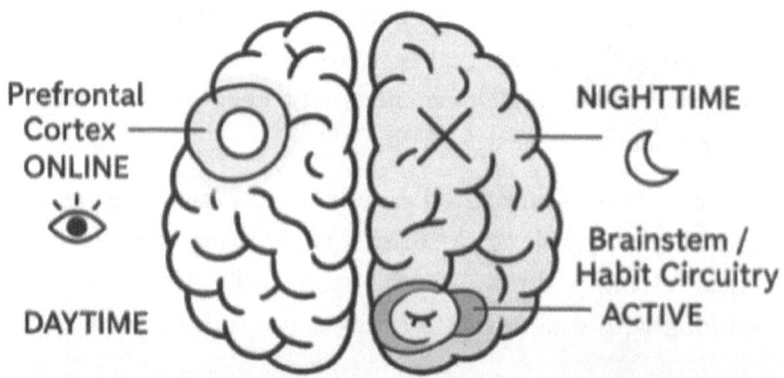

This explains an important contrast. While awake, you can notice early tension, respond to biofeedback, adjust posture, or soften your breath. During sleep, there is no referee watching the play. The jaw responds to signals without oversight.

If the nervous system senses arousal, airway compromise, or unresolved load, the jaw may brace reflexively.

This is not a failure of discipline. It is a shift in governance. Sleep places the jaw under automatic control, where old habits and protective reflexes dominate. Understanding this removes blame and clarifies strategy. You cannot rely on willpower at night. You must work with the systems that remain active.

2) Loss of conscious feedback allows force to escalate

In waking life, the body relies heavily on sensory feedback to prevent self-injury. If you bite down too hard on a fork or clench excessively during the day, pain receptors and periodontal ligaments send immediate signals to the brain that reduce force. These feedback loops act as natural governors.[5]

During sleep, those protective loops are dampened. Sensory thresholds rise, pain processing changes, and conscious awareness is offline. As a result, the jaw can generate forces far beyond what you would ever allow while awake.[9]

Sleep-related clenching and grinding episodes can involve extremely high bite forces, sometimes described in the range of 200 to 250 pounds or more at the molars in severe cases.[9]

These contractions can also be sustained for several seconds and repeated dozens of times in a single night. The precise number is less important than the principle. Sleep removes the stop signal. Without feedback and correction, the jaw can press harder, longer, and more frequently than it ever would under conscious control.

Muscles fatigue, teeth absorb load, and joint structures experience repeated stress, all without the person knowing it is happening.

This is why people often wake with jaw soreness, headaches, or a heavy facial feeling despite having no memory of clenching.5 The damage accumulates quietly. Recognizing that sleep physiology permits force escalation is critical.

It explains why protection matters at night and why daytime retraining alone is often insufficient.

3) Micro-arousals are the engine behind sleep jaw activity

Most sleep-related bruxism does not occur as a continuous grind throughout the night. Instead, it appears in bursts that are closely linked to brief sleep disruptions known as micro-arousals.

Micro-arousals are short, involuntary shifts in brain activity that typically last between three and fifteen seconds. You usually do not remember them, and they are not full awakenings, but they are enough to activate alerting systems.

When a micro-arousal occurs, the nervous system briefly shifts toward a sympathetic state. Heart rate rises. Brain waves move toward wake-like patterns. Motor systems receive a surge of activation. In this window, the brainstem may trigger rhythmic or sustained jaw muscle activity, known clinically as Rhythmic Masticatory Muscle Activity, or RMMA.

RMMA can present as clenching, grinding, or subtle chewing-like movements. It is not random. It is a patterned motor response tied to arousal. Factors that increase the frequency of micro-arousals, such as stress carryover, airway instability, pain, noise, alcohol, caffeine, or irregular sleep schedules, also increase the likelihood of jaw activity.

In simple terms, micro-arousals are the match, and jaw activation is the flame. Reduce the arousals, and the fire has less fuel. This insight shifts the focus from the jaw alone to the broader sleep and nervous system environment that drives it.

Airway instability: when clenching is a stabilization reflex

One of the most common drivers of sleep bruxism events is the body's attempt to protect breathing.[6,8] As sleep deepens, throat and tongue tone decreases.[7,8] If the airway narrows, because of sleep position, nasal obstruction, alcohol, congestion, or undiagnosed sleep-disordered breathing, the brain may interpret that narrowing as threat.[6,8]

In response, the body recruits the jaw as an anchor:

a forceful clench can stabilize the mandible.

forward jaw movement can help open the airway.

the brain prioritizes breathing over teeth.

This is why, for many people, nighttime clenching is not merely a "bad habit." It can be a survival reflex that happens to be tooth-damaging.[6,8]

This is also why persistent sleep bruxism should raise a clinical question: what is fragmenting sleep or destabilizing the airway?[7,8]

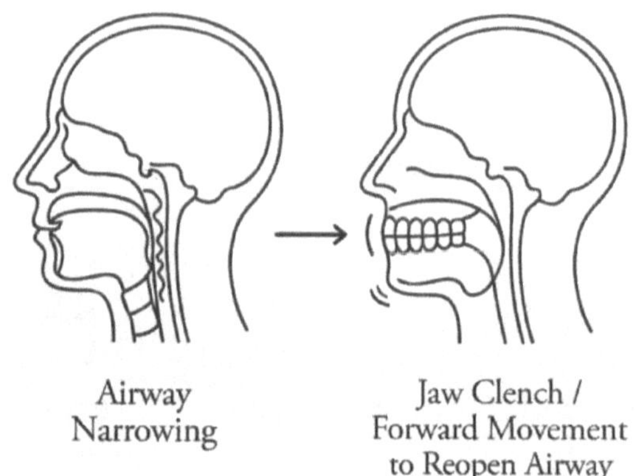

Airway
Narrowing

Jaw Clench /
Forward Movement
to Reopen Airway

Light, screens, and the "melatonin gap"

Light exposure, especially evening exposure to bright LEDs and screens, can keep the nervous system in a higher arousal state into the night.[11,13]

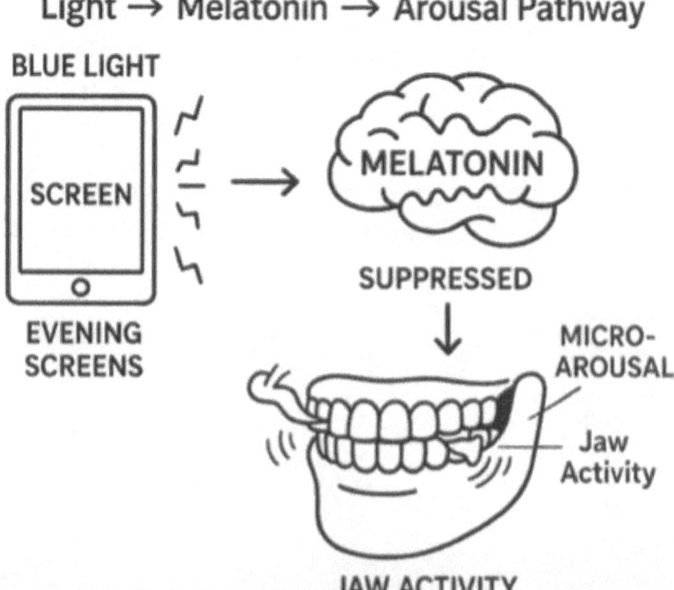

The pathway in plain terms

Evening light suppresses melatonin signaling and delays the body's shift into sleep physiology.[11,13] When melatonin is delayed, the nervous system often remains more reactive.[4,5,11,12]

More reactivity means a lower threshold for micro-arousals. More micro-arousals means more RMMA bursts and more jaw activity.[4,5] This is why late-night scrolling frequently correlates with:

- o lighter, more "brittle" sleep more awakenings (even if you do not remember them)
- o more morning jaw fatigue or tooth soreness. [11,12]

The day-to-night transition: your "stress bucket" echoes in sleep

Nighttime clenching is often the echo of daytime load. If your nervous system never fully downshifts during the day, high cognitive load, constant stimulation, unresolved tension, then you tend to enter sleep with elevated baseline arousal.

That state does not prevent sleep, but it makes sleep more fragile. Fragile sleep produces more micro-arousals. Micro-arousals produce more jaw events. A useful mindset: you do not eliminate nighttime clenching by forcing the jaw to behave. You reduce it by lowering the system's need to spike.

BRUX at night: what you can control vs. what you protect

Night requires two parallel strategies:

1) Protect against involuntary force

Because you cannot "train" yourself while asleep, passive protection matters. A passive guard can help distribute forces and reduce direct tooth-on-tooth damage on nights when events occur.[10]

2) Engineer fewer triggers

This is the BRUX Method applied to sleep:

B — Build Awareness: identify what worsens night clenching (screens, alcohol, congestion, stress spikes, snoring, waking with dry mouth)

R — Relax the Response: downshift the nervous system before sleep

U — Understand Triggers: track the specific inputs that create brittle sleep

X — eXchange the Pattern: replace late stimulation with a repeatable wind-down loop

A practical wind-down routine for nighttime clenching

Use this as a default "quiet the arousal centers" sequence. It is designed to reduce micro-arousal likelihood and lower jaw muscle readiness.

60 minutes before bed: reduce stimulation

Dim lights; avoid bright overhead LEDs

If you must use screens, lower brightness and reduce visual intensity (larger text, fewer rapid inputs)

10 minutes before bed: shift physiology

4–7–8 breathing or any extended-exhale practice

Brief jaw release: lips together, teeth apart, tongue to the palate

Gentle shoulder drop on each exhale

At lights out: protect and stabilize

If you use a passive guard, this is when it earns its keep

Prioritize nasal breathing cues (lip seal, tongue posture) to support airway stability

What to watch for: signs your night clenching is not just "stress"

Nighttime clenching becomes clinically meaningful when it clusters with airway and sleep fragmentation signs, such as:

- loud snoring, gasping, or witnessed breathing pauses
- waking with dry mouth or sore throat
- morning headaches that fade after getting up
- persistent daytime sleepiness despite "enough hours"
- significant tooth wear, fractures, or repeated restorations breaking

Those patterns suggest you may be seeing micro-arousal load, and potentially airway-driven stabilization clenching, a different category than simple habit.

The Goal is not Perfect Stillness. It is a Quieter Night.
Nighttime clenching is automatic. It is not a moral failing, and it is not a discipline problem. It is physiology. When you fall asleep, the part of the brain that does conscious inhibition and self-monitoring goes offline.

The body is then guided by autonomic rhythms, brief arousal spikes, and protective reflexes. If your nervous system is running hot from the day, if your sleep is fragile, or if your airway becomes unstable, the jaw may activate the way it was designed to activate as a stabilizer, a bracing tool, and sometimes an emergency response.

That framing matters because it changes your strategy. If you treat nighttime clenching like a character flaw, you will reach for willpower, self-criticism, and force. None of those are available during sleep. If you treat it like a systems issue, you start working with reality.

You stop trying to control the night directly and start shaping the conditions that make the night less reactive. A mature, realistic plan has three layers. First, reduce the triggers you can control.

Light and stimulation set your arousal threshold. Late-night screens, bright overhead lighting, and constant input keep the brain in a state of readiness when it should be downshifting. Stress carryover does the same thing.

If your body goes to bed still "solving" the day, the nervous system stays closer to the surface, and micro-arousals become easier to trigger. Your aim is not an elaborate routine. Your aim is a clean transition.

Lower stimulation, lower light, and lower the need to stay on guard.

Second, protect the teeth during the hours you cannot control. Sleep is not the time for negotiations with your nervous system. If clenching occurs, the priority is to reduce damage.

A protective night guard distributes force and reduces the risk of wear, chipping, cracking, and joint irritation.[10] This is not surrender. It is risk management. It is what responsible care looks like when the forces are involuntary and the bite can become stronger than anything you would choose while awake.

Third, train the system during the day so the night has less residual motor excitation to express. Nighttime bruxism is often an echo of daytime load. When you reduce daytime bracing, you reduce the baseline tone of the jaw muscles and lower the overall arousal level that carries into sleep. [15]

This is where biofeedback and skill-building matter.[14,15] Daytime training does not eliminate every night event, but it changes the terrain. The nervous system becomes less reactive. Sleep becomes more stable. The jaw has fewer reasons to fire.

When you approach sleep clenching as a whole-system pattern rather than a jaw-only problem, the goal becomes clear. You are not chasing perfect stillness. You are building a quieter night.

Over time, that looks like deeper sleep, fewer micro-arousals, less sympathetic "spiking," and a jaw that no longer has to brace in the dark to keep you safe.

References

Sleep neurobiology, inhibition, and "offline" executive control

1. Braun AR, Balkin TJ, Wesenten NJ, et al. Regional cerebral blood flow throughout the sleep-wake cycle: an H2(15)O PET study. Brain. 1997;120(7):1173-1197. doi:10.1093/brain/120.7.1173

2. Maquet P. The role of sleep in learning and memory. Science. 2001;294(5544):1048-1052. doi:10.1126/science.1062856

Micro-arousals, RMMA, and sleep bruxism event physiology

3. American Academy of Sleep Medicine. The AASM Manual for the Scoring of Sleep and Associated Events: Rules, Terminology and Technical Specifications. Darien, IL: American Academy of Sleep Medicine; 2020.

4. Kato T, Rompré PH, Montplaisir JY, Sessle BJ, Lavigne GJ. Sleep bruxism: an oromotor activity secondary to micro-arousal. J Dent Res. 2001;80(10):1940-1944. doi:10.1177/00220345010800101501

5. Lavigne GJ, Khoury S, Abe S, Yamaguchi T, Raphael K. Bruxism physiology and pathology: an overview for clinicians. J Oral Rehabil. 2008;35(7):476-494. doi:10.1111/j.1365-2842.2008.01881.x

Sleep-disordered breathing and airway-related arousal contributions

6. Khoury S, Rouleau GA, Rompré PH, Mayer P, Montplaisir JY, Lavigne GJ. A significant increase in breathing amplitude precedes sleep bruxism. Chest. 2008;134(2):332-337. doi:10.1378/chest.07-2317

7. Carra MC, Huynh N, Lavigne GJ. Sleep bruxism: a comprehensive overview for the dental clinician interested in sleep medicine. Dent Clin North Am. 2012;56(2):387-413. doi:10.1016/j.cden.2012.01.003

8. Balasubramaniam R, Klasser GD, Cistulli PA, Lavigne GJ. The link between sleep bruxism, sleep disordered breathing, and temporomandibular disorders: an evidence-based review. J Dent Sleep Med. 2014;1(1):27-37.

Force generation during sleep bruxism and why protection is used

9. Nishigawa K, Bando E, Nakano M. Quantitative study of bite force during sleep associated bruxism. J Oral Rehabil. 2001;28(5):485-491.

10. Jagger RG, Korszun A. The effectiveness of occlusal splints for sleep bruxism. Br Dent J. 2008;205(10):E19.

Evening light, screens, melatonin timing, and sleep/circadian effects

11. Chang AM, Aeschbach D, Duffy JF, Czeisler CA. Evening use of light-emitting eReaders negatively affects sleep, circadian timing, and next-morning alertness. Proc Natl Acad Sci U S A. 2015;112(4):1232-1237. doi:10.1073/pnas.1418490112

12. Cajochen C, Frey S, Anders D, et al. Evening exposure to a light-emitting diodes (LED)-backlit computer screen affects circadian physiology and cognitive performance. J Appl Physiol (1985). 2011;110(5):1432-1438. doi:10.1152/japplphysiol.00165.2011

13. Brainard GC, Hanifin JP, Greeson JM, et al. Action spectrum for melatonin regulation in humans: evidence for a novel circadian photoreceptor. J Neurosci.

2001;21(16):6405-6412. doi:10.1523/JNEUROSCI.21-16-06405.2001

Biofeedback as contingent feedback supporting operant learning (mechanism-level support)

14. Ilovar S, Džunková M, Kovač Z, et al. Biofeedback for treatment of awake and sleep bruxism in adults. Syst Rev. 2014;3:42. doi:10.1186/2046-4053-3-42

15. de Albuquerque Vieira M, Moreira VG, da Silva MA, et al. Effectiveness of biofeedback in individuals with awake bruxism: a systematic review. Medicina (Kaunas). 2023;59(2):—. (Open-access systematic review in PMC.)

Part IV:
Restore: Supporting the Biology

How internal physiology shapes muscle tone, mood and resilience.

Meet Carly.

Carly was a 34-year-old marketing executive who lived inside a stream of inputs. Her smartwatch vibrated fifty times a day, her phone another hundred. She joked that she worked one notification at a time, as if attention were just another KPI to optimize.

Even her "breaks" were filled with scrolling, quick replies, and checking what she might have missed. By late afternoon, her body told a different story. A steady ache gathered behind her temples, and her jaw felt dense and overworked, like it had been holding tension on assignment. Some evenings she noticed soreness in the muscles on the sides of her face or a tight band across her across her forehead.

She never remembered clenching, not once, but her dentist showed her the evidence: flattened cusps, early gum recession, and a wear pattern that did not require audible grinding to do real damage. Carly tried the usual fixes because they felt logical. She adjusted her chair, bought a better pillow, swapped coffee for tea, promised herself she would "relax more," and even tried stretching her neck between meetings.

Nothing stuck, because the trigger was not one dramatic stressor. It was the constant switching, the micro-urgency of being perpetually on call. Her nervous system never truly downshifted, and her jaw, as always, volunteered to brace so the rest of her system could keep performing. One Saturday, her phone died during a hike. The first hour felt itchy, like she was ignoring something important. The second hour felt oddly spacious. By the third, she noticed a small, unfamiliar sensation: her jaw had softened without her trying.

Her shoulders dropped. Her breath moved lower. That weekend became her first digital detox, not as a self-improvement trend, but as a muscle experiment. For the first time, she could feel the direct link between stimulation and bracing, and she finally had a path forward based on cause, not guesswork.

Chapter 11: Hormones, Hydration, and Muscle Tone

Jaw clenching does not occur in isolation from the rest of the body. Hormones and hydration quietly shape the background conditions in which your nervous system operates. When these internal regulators shift, the baseline tone of your muscles shifts with them.

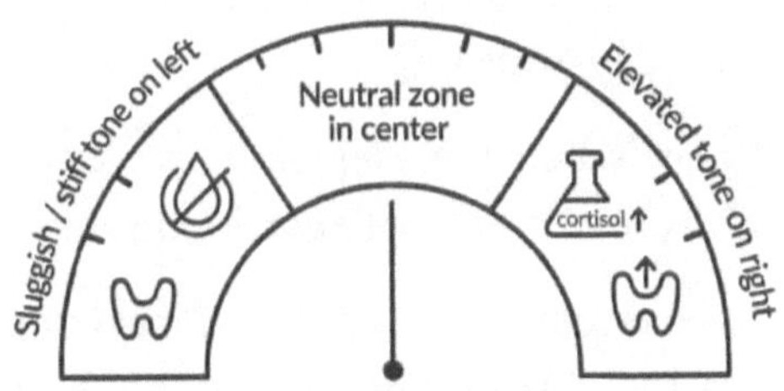

When these internal regulators shift,
the baseline tone of your muscles shifts
with them.

For many people, this explains why clenching can intensify even when stress levels or daily routines have not obviously changed. This chapter explains how hormonal signals and fluid balance influence muscle tone, pain sensitivity, and jaw activity, and how to work with these systems rather than fight them.

Hormones as Regulators of Muscle Tone

Hormones act as chemical messengers that influence how excitable your nervous system is at rest. When hormone levels fluctuate, the electrical threshold that controls muscle contraction changes. The jaw muscles are particularly sensitive to these shifts because they are tightly linked to the autonomic nervous system and to stress regulation.

173

Rather than thinking of clenching as a purely behavioral issue, it is more accurate to view it as a response that is amplified or dampened by hormonal context.

Cortisol: The High Alert Signal

Cortisol is the hormone most closely associated with stress and survival readiness.[1,2] Its purpose is to mobilize energy, sharpen vigilance, and prepare the body for action, not restoration. In healthy rhythm, cortisol rises in the morning to help you wake, then gradually declines as the day ends.[2]

Problems begin when that signal stays elevated into the evening or remains high across weeks of sustained pressure.

When cortisol remains elevated, the nervous system behaves as if danger is nearby.[1,2] Motor neurons become more electrically active, which makes muscles easier to recruit and harder to quiet.[1] For the jaw, that often means the masseter and temporalis carry a higher resting tone.

You may not feel an obvious clench, but the system is braced. Teeth contact becomes more likely, and the threshold for clenching drops. Smaller triggers, a difficult email, a tense conversation, a traffic delay, can produce a stronger jaw response because the body is already primed.

This is why many people notice increased clenching during prolonged stress, disrupted sleep, illness, pain flare-ups, or emotional strain. The jaw is not "misbehaving." It is following a body-wide chemical instruction that says: stay ready.

Over time, chronically elevated cortisol can prevent a full return to neutral baseline. Even during downtime, the jaw may remain subtly activated, as if it is standing guard. The practical implication is simple.

Lowering the overall stress signal, especially in the day-to-night transition, makes it easier for the jaw to soften without force.

Estrogen and Progesterone: The Cyclical Effect

For many individuals, jaw tension follows a predictable rhythm that mirrors hormonal changes across the menstrual cycle and through life stages such as perimenopause and menopause.

This is not imagined, and it is not purely psychological. Estrogen and progesterone influence muscle elasticity, connective tissue behavior, joint lubrication, and pain perception.[3,5] When these signals shift, the baseline "tone" of the jaw system can shift with them.

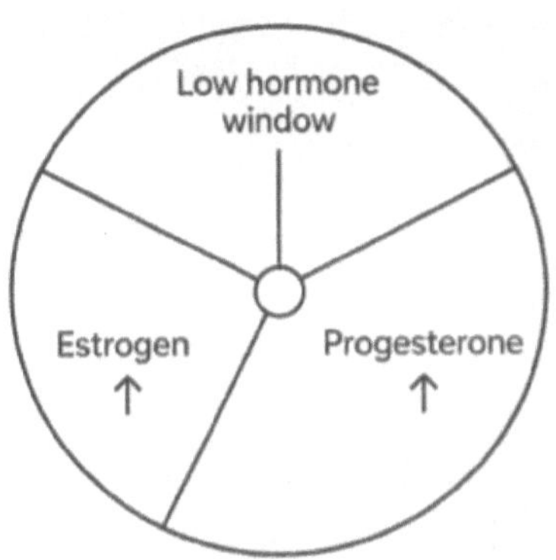

A common pattern appears in the days leading up to menstruation, when estrogen and progesterone drop.[4] During this window, many people report increased jaw stiffness, facial fatigue, and a lower threshold for headache or TMJ soreness.

The same mechanical load that felt tolerable two weeks earlier can suddenly feel sharp or exhausting. One reason is that hormonal decline can increase pain sensitivity and reduce the feeling of cushioning in tissues that normally tolerate micro-stress.

Progesterone plays a calming role for many bodies.[6] When progesterone is low, stress reactivity tends to rise. The nervous system becomes easier to activate, and muscle bracing becomes more likely. In practical terms, the jaw is more prone to "holding" during

175

concentration, conflict, or emotional load, even when the external stressor is modest.

Estrogen also has direct relevance to the jaw joint. The temporomandibular joint and surrounding tissues have a high density of estrogen receptors, which means the TMJ can be unusually responsive to hormonal fluctuation.[3]

During periods of low estrogen, the joint can feel drier, less cushioned, and more reactive. In that state, clenching tends to feel more painful and more fatiguing, not because you are doing more, but because the system is less buffered.

Testosterone and Muscle Intensity

Testosterone influences muscle strength, recovery capacity, and tissue repair, including in the masticatory system.[7,8] When testosterone levels are higher, the jaw muscles, especially the masseter and temporalis, tend to be stronger and capable of generating greater bite force. [8]

That can be an advantage for normal function like chewing. However, it also means that when clenching occurs, the load transferred into teeth, restorations, and the temporomandibular joints can be substantially higher than the person would ever apply consciously. The habit may be subtle, but the mechanical impact can be significant. Testosterone also supports the body's ability to recover from muscular work. Clenching is an isometric contraction that creates metabolic demand and produces byproducts that the body must clear.

When recovery systems are robust, the jaw can return to baseline more quickly after a stressful day or a night with elevated motor activity. As testosterone gradually declines with age, the recovery side of the equation often changes first.[7] Muscle repair tends to slow.

Lactic acid and inflammatory byproducts may clear less efficiently. Tissues can feel more "sticky" and reactive, and jaw soreness may linger longer after clenching episodes. This is one reason people sometimes report that their jaw tension feels heavier or more fatiguing over time.

The key point is that increasing discomfort does not necessarily mean the behavior is worsening. It can reflect a shift in physiology: similar clenching, slower recovery, and a higher cost for the same habit.

Thyroid Hormones and Baseline Tension

Thyroid hormones help regulate how quickly your body uses energy and how responsive your muscles are throughout the day.[9] When these hormones are out of balance, many people notice changes in overall tension, restlessness, or stiffness. This matters for bruxism because jaw muscles are already sensitive to stress, focus, and emotional load.

When thyroid activity is higher than usual, people often describe feeling keyed up or unable to fully relax.[9] Muscles may feel more alert even during rest. This heightened neuromuscular activity can make it harder to keep your jaw in a neutral position.

You may notice subtle clenching while concentrating, driving, or scrolling, even if you are not feeling emotionally stressed.

When thyroid activity is lower, the experience can be different but still challenging. Muscles may feel tight, heavy, or slow to recover after use.[10] Jaw fatigue can linger longer after chewing or speaking. Stiffness can increase background tension, making relaxed jaw posture feel unfamiliar or effortful.

In both situations, the common thread is elevated baseline tension. Your jaw muscles start the day closer to activation than rest. From a CBT perspective, this does not mean something is wrong with you.

177

It means your nervous system may need clearer cues to recognize when clenching is happening and when release is possible.

Biofeedback can support this awareness. Tools like ClenchAlert provide a gentle signal when clenching begins, helping you notice tension earlier rather than after pain appears. Over time, this repeated feedback supports habit change.

You practice returning your jaw to rest, even when your body's baseline tension is higher than usual. The goal is not to force relaxation. It is to build awareness, respond intentionally, and make neutral jaw posture easier to access throughout your day.

Hydration and Muscle Reactivity

Hydration affects how your muscles contract, relax, and recover.[11,12] Even mild dehydration can change the way your nervous system and muscle fibers behave. If you live with chronic clenching or grinding, this can matter more than you expect because your jaw muscles tend to run "on" by default.

When your body is low on fluids, electrolyte balance becomes less stable.[11,12] Electrolytes help regulate nerve signaling and muscle firing. When that system is off, muscles can feel jumpy, tight, or slower to release. You may also fatigue faster.[13] A muscle that tires quickly is more likely to hold tension, especially during long stretches of focus, stress, or screen time. Your jaw muscles are no exception. Dehydration can make clenching feel stronger and more uncomfortable. It can also make your jaw harder to "let go" once you notice tension. Many people recognize this pattern late in the day, when they have been busy, talking, sipping coffee, and forgetting plain water.[11,12]

By evening, the jaw feels tight, your bite feels heavy, and relaxing your face takes more effort than it should. From a CBT-informed perspective, hydration is a supportive condition, not a cure. You are reducing background friction so your habit change tools work better. When your body is well hydrated, muscle firing tends to be smoother, and your nervous system can downshift more easily.

Biofeedback can help you catch dehydration-related clenching early. A device like ClenchAlert can prompt awareness the moment you start to clamp down, which gives you a chance to reset your jaw, take a breath, and choose a different response. Pair that cue with a simple habit, like drinking a glass of water, and you reinforce a calmer baseline over time.[14,15]

The goal is consistency. Small, steady hydration habits can make relaxed jaw posture easier to access throughout the day.

Summary: Hormonal and Physiological Influences on the Jaw

Factor	Primary Effect on Muscle Tone	Jaw Impact
High Cortisol	Increased motor neuron excitability	Persistent bracing and clenching
Low Estrogen	Reduced joint lubrication and higher pain sensitivity	Stiffness and TMJ discomfort
Low Progesterone	Reduced muscle relaxation	Heightened daytime clenching
Testosterone Shifts	Changes in muscle force and recovery	Stronger or longer-lasting soreness
Poor Hydration	Increased muscle irritability	Faster fatigue and tighter jaw

Managing Hormonal and Hydration-Related Clenching

You cannot eliminate hormonal fluctuations, but you can reduce their impact on your jaw.

Practical strategies include:

- Tracking patterns to identify weeks or seasons when clenching worsens
- Using awareness tools like the ClenchAlert Active Guard more consistently during high-risk windows

- Supporting muscle relaxation with adequate hydration and electrolyte balance
- Using warmth to increase blood flow to the jaw during periods of stiffness
- Prioritizing sleep and breathing practices that reduce cortisol before bedtime

These approaches do not override hormones. They help buffer their effects so the jaw does not carry the full burden of internal change.

Fluid, Fuel, and Muscle Tone

Hormones and hydration quietly set the stage on which jaw clenching plays out. They influence the nervous system long before you notice a thought, a deadline, or a trigger.

When cortisol is elevated, the body behaves as if it must stay ready. Muscle tone rises, the stress threshold drops, and the jaw becomes an easy place for that vigilance to land. When estrogen and progesterone shift, pain sensitivity and tissue reactivity can change, and the jaw joint and chewing muscles may feel less forgiving, more inflamed, or simply more prone to guarding. When testosterone and thyroid function vary, recovery capacity and baseline muscle stiffness can change as well.

None of this means you are doing something wrong. It means your system is receiving different internal instructions, and the jaw is responding exactly as a protective system would.

Hydration adds another layer because fluid balance affects how muscles contract and release. When you are underhydrated, tissues can feel "sticky," fatigue shows up faster, and small amounts of tension may linger instead of clearing.

Electrolyte balance matters too, because nerve signaling and muscle relaxation rely on minerals that help regulate excitability. In practical

181

terms, a day with low water intake, high caffeine, poor sleep, or heavy stress can create the perfect internal conditions for clenching to feel stronger and harder to interrupt.

This is why progress can feel inconsistent even when your effort is steady. The inputs changed, so the output changed. The goal of this chapter is not to turn clenching into a chemistry project or to make you track every variable. It is to expand your model.

When you understand that biology influences muscle tone, you stop blaming yourself for fluctuation and you start responding with skill.

That response can be simple: drink water before you are thirsty, add electrolytes when needed, reduce the evening cortisol slope with a longer exhale, and use warmth or gentle movement when stiffness is high.

If you notice cyclical patterns, plan for them by using more support during high risk windows rather than waiting for pain to force your attention. This is the deeper takeaway: you cannot always control hormones, but you can control your interpretation of their effects.

Awareness reduces urgency, and reduced urgency lowers threat. When you pair that awareness with hydration and gentle regulation, you change the internal environment that makes clenching feel necessary. The jaw does not have to fight biology. It only needs enough safety and support to return to its neutral resting state, even while the body is shifting.

References

Hormones as regulators of arousal, stress physiology, and muscle tone (cortisol)

1. O'Byrne NA, Ainsworth B, Semple S, Ovens J, Gable D, Atkinson L. Understanding the relationship between stress and musculoskeletal pain: a narrative review. Ir J Med Sci. 2021;190(1):105-116.

2. Andreadi A, Tsiakou A, Filippou C, et al. The cortisol awakening response: a systematic review and meta-analysis. Psychoneuroendocrinology. 2025;165:106979.

Sex hormones and the jaw system (estrogen/progesterone; pain sensitivity; TMJ receptor biology)

3. Robinson JL, Cass K, Aronson K, et al. Estrogen and the temporomandibular joint: a review of the literature. J Oral Rehabil. 2019;46(4):339-351.

4. LeResche L, Mancl LA, Sherman JJ, Gandara B, Dworkin SF. Changes in temporomandibular pain and other symptoms across the menstrual cycle. Pain. 2003;106(3):253-261.

5. Zieliński G, Sierpińska T, Lipski M. Estrogen levels and temporomandibular disorders: a systematic review. Int J Environ Res Public Health. 2024;21(4):482.

6. Kapur J, Joshi S. Neurosteroids and their therapeutic potential in anxiety and stress-related disorders. Curr Opin Pharmacol. 2021;60:22-30.

Testosterone, muscle capacity, force, and recovery with age

7. Bhasin S, Brito JP, Cunningham GR, et al. Testosterone therapy in men with hypogonadism: an Endocrine Society clinical practice guideline. J Clin Endocrinol Metab. 2018;103(5):1715-1744.

8. Palinkas M, Nassar MS, Cecílio FA, et al. Age and gender influence on maximal bite force and masticatory muscles thickness. Arch Oral Biol. 2010;55(10):797-802.

Thyroid hormones and neuromuscular responsiveness, stiffness, and fatigue

9. Salvatore D, Simonides WS, Dentice M, Zavacki AM, Larsen PR. Thyroid hormones and skeletal muscle—new insights and potential implications. Nat Rev Endocrinol. 2014;10(4):206-214.

10. Sindoni A, Rodolico C, Pappalardo MA, et al. Hypothyroid myopathy: a peculiar clinical presentation of thyroid failure. Review. Endocrine. 2016;52(2):339-345.

Hydration, electrolytes, neuromuscular function, and fatigue

11. McDermott BP, Anderson SA, Armstrong LE, et al. National Athletic Trainers' Association position statement: fluid replacement for the physically active. J Athl Train. 2017;52(9):877-895.

12. Francisco R, Antunes B, Mota J, et al. Does acute dehydration affect neuromuscular function? A systematic review. Appl Physiol Nutr Metab. 2024;49(10):1043-1056.

13. Barley OR, Chapman DW, Abbiss CR. Acute dehydration impairs endurance without modulating neuromuscular function. Front Physiol. 2018;9:1562.

Biofeedback as a learning mechanism (operant learning; awareness-to-response coupling)

14. Schwartz MS, Andrasik F, eds. Biofeedback: A Practitioner's Guide. 4th ed. New York, NY: Guilford Press; 2017.

15. Manfredini D, Ahlberg J, Aarab G, et al. Awake bruxism: systematic review of current evidence and clinical management. J Oral Rehabil. 2019;46(5):448-461.

Chapter 12: Pain, Protection, and the Nervous System

Pain is supposed to be protective. In most parts of the body, pain teaches avoidance. Touch a hot surface and your hand pulls away. With the jaw, the opposite often happens.

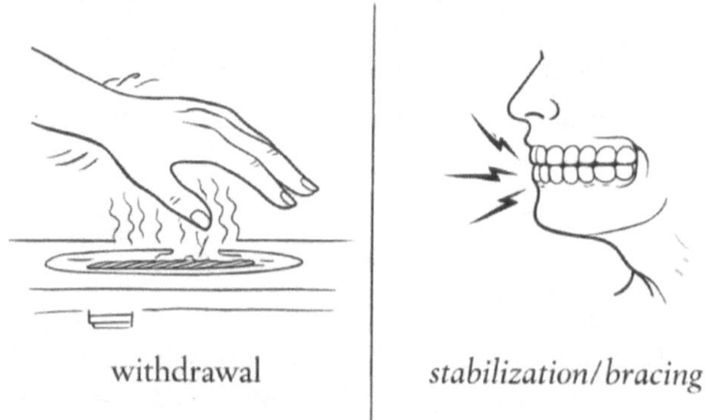

Pain does not stop clenching. It reinforces it. This is not a failure of willpower or awareness. It is a predictable response of the nervous system when it interprets jaw discomfort as a structural threat rather than a local injury. Once this protective logic is activated, the body enters a loop where pain and tension continually amplify one another.

Understanding this loop is essential, because trying to fight jaw pain with effort almost always makes it worse.

Why Jaw Pain Triggers More Clenching

When the nervous system detects pain in the jaw or temporomandibular joint, it does not respond with withdrawal. Instead, it responds with stabilization.[1,2] From the brain's perspective,

186

the jaw is not a fingertip. It is a load-bearing structure that anchors the skull, airway, and cervical spine.

When something in that system hurts, the brain's priority becomes immobilization. This creates what is known as the pain–spasm–pain cycle.[1,2]

The Splinting Reflex

When jaw pain shows up, your nervous system often responds with splinting. Splinting is a protective strategy: the brain tries to prevent further irritation by holding a body part as still as possible. In the jaw, that "stillness" is created by sending a steady contraction signal to the masseter and temporalis muscles.

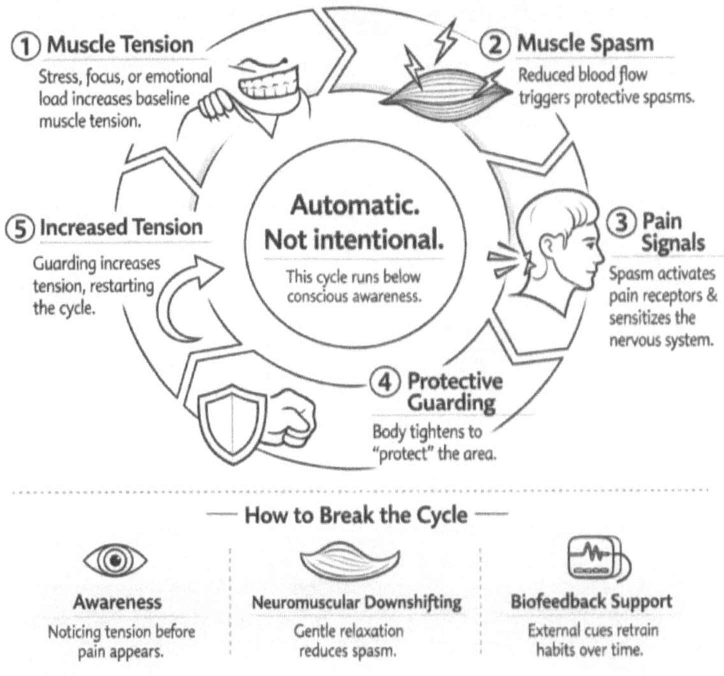

The practical result is sustained clenching.

This is where the cycle becomes self-defeating. The brain is attempting to reduce pain by stabilizing the jaw, but the stabilization method is the same motor pattern that often contributes to the pain in the first place.

As the muscles stay contracted, blood flow is restricted and oxygen delivery drops. The tissue begins to fatigue, and metabolic byproducts accumulate. That combination can increase sensitivity and amplify soreness.

When discomfort rises, the nervous system often interprets it as a sign of ongoing threat, so it doubles down on the "protective" strategy and increases muscle guarding.

The jaw feels tighter, relief becomes harder to access, and the pain signal becomes more persistent. Over time, splinting can turn an acute flare into a repeating pain-tension loop.[1,2,5]

Central Sensitization and the Stuck Volume Knob

When jaw pain lasts long enough, your nervous system can adapt in a way that makes it more reactive, not more resilient. This shift is often described as central sensitization.[3,4]

Instead of the body "getting used to" pain and calming down, the brain and spinal

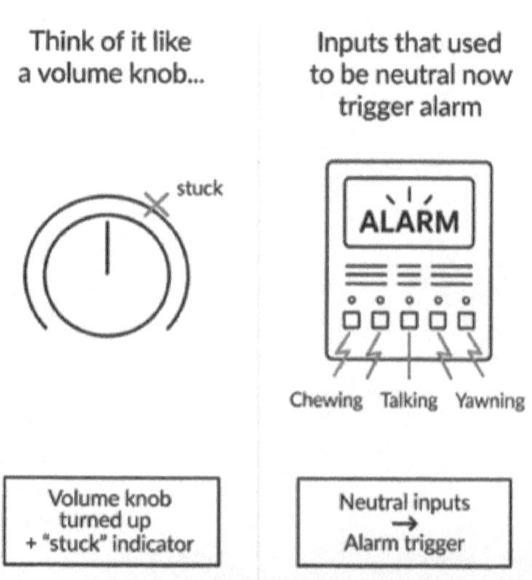

cord begin treating jaw-related input as higher priority.

Think of it like a volume knob that has been turned up and then gets stuck there. With repeated pain signals, the nervous system's gain control changes. Nerves that once needed strong stimulation to fire may begin responding to much smaller cues. Sensations that used to feel neutral, like light tooth contact, normal jaw movement, chewing, or even holding your mouth still, can start to register as danger.

Stress, fatigue, poor sleep, or prolonged concentration can add more background activation and make the system even easier to trigger. In this phase, clenching can become less of a reaction and more of a default posture.

Your brain is not necessarily waiting for a clear threat. It is using muscle tension as a constant "brace," because tension feels like protection. [2,3,4] Over time, this posture can persist even when the original injury or flare has improved. A common trap here is misreading the signal. Many people assume their jaw is relaxed because the sharp, obvious pain has faded.

But the absence of sharp pain does not always mean the muscles are quiet. Instead, the sensory map can become less precise. Tension becomes familiar, baseline effort fades into the background, and your nervous system continues running a protective program you no longer consciously notice.

The Sympathetic Loop

Pain does not stay local. When jaw pain rises, it reliably activates the sympathetic nervous system, the same system that prepares you for urgency and threat. Your brain reads pain as a signal that something is wrong and responds by releasing stress chemistry, including adrenaline and cortisol.

These chemicals increase baseline muscle tone, heighten vigilance, and shift your body into an "action-ready" state. In that state,

189

relaxation is not simply a choice. It becomes physiologically difficult, even if you want it.

This is how the loop forms.

Pain increases stress chemistry. Stress chemistry increases muscle bracing. Muscle bracing increases pain.[1,2,5,6] In the jaw, bracing often shows up as clenching, tongue tension, facial tightness, and rigid posture through the neck and shoulders. Even low-level clenching can keep the muscles active long enough to reduce blood flow, accelerate fatigue, and create chemical irritation in the tissue.

That irritation feeds more pain input back into the nervous system, which the brain interprets as confirmation that more protection is needed. The sympathetic system stays online, and the cycle tightens.

Once this loop is established, telling yourself to relax usually fails for a simple reason: the nervous system is not prioritizing comfort. It is prioritizing safety. A "calm down" command cannot override a brain that believes it must stay on guard.

That is why willpower-based strategies often feel discouraging in this phase. The more effective approach is to work with the system rather than argue with it. You interrupt the loop by adding small safety cues and short releases that the nervous system can tolerate, then repeating them consistently until bracing no longer feels necessary.

Over time, the body learns that downshifting is safe, and tension stops being the default.

Why Pain Is a Poor Teacher for the Jaw

Pain is an effective teacher when the correct response is simple: pull away. Touch a hot stove, and you withdraw. The lesson is clear, the movement is automatic, and the system calms once the threat is gone. The jaw does not work that way.

When the brain detects jaw pain, it rarely chooses "withdrawal." It chooses stability. The nervous system treats the jaw like a structure that must be held in place to prevent further damage. That decision drives co-contraction and splinting, meaning multiple jaw muscles stay active at the same time to brace the joint. Instead of letting the area soften, the system tightens.

This changes the learning outcome. With most injuries, pain teaches avoidance and reduces exposure. With jaw pain, pain can teach the opposite: it increases guarding, raises baseline muscle tone, and keeps the body in a fight-or-flight state.

Over time, repeated pain input can also increase sensitivity, so the threshold for bracing drops. Clenching becomes easier to trigger and harder to notice. That is why "waiting until it hurts enough to stop" often fails.

Pain does not reveal the habit. It can convert the habit into a reflex. You may clench to protect the jaw, then the clenching adds more muscle fatigue and irritation, which the brain reads as more danger, which drives more bracing.

If you want less clenching, pain is not the cue to rely on. You need earlier signals and deliberate interruption strategies, before the nervous system locks into protection mode.

How the Nervous System Learns Protective Tension

Protective jaw tension is not random. It is learned through a process called sensory-motor association. When your nervous system detects pain, strain, or perceived threat in the jaw, the amygdala flags danger and signals the brainstem to increase muscle readiness. This increases muscle spindle activity in the jaw closers, causing the muscles to shorten and stiffen. The goal is simple: limit movement to protect the structure. If the threat is brief, this response can resolve.

When the threat persists, however, the pathway is reinforced through repetition. The brain learns that clenching equals safety. Over time, this learning is strengthened through long-term potentiation, meaning the signal becomes faster, stronger, and easier to trigger. The amount of input required to activate clenching drops. Eventually, the jaw may brace even when pain is mild or no longer present.

This process is compounded by sensory-motor amnesia. When a muscle remains partially contracted for long periods, the brain gradually stops recognizing that contraction as abnormal. Tension becomes the new baseline. Clenching feels neutral. Teeth touching feels ordinary.

You may believe your jaw is relaxed when, physiologically, it is still active. At this stage, internal awareness alone is often unreliable. Because the nervous system has normalized tension, you cannot accurately feel when clenching starts. External feedback becomes necessary to reveal the habit and create opportunities for interruption before the system escalates into full guarding.

Why Chronic Pain Keeps the Jaw on Guard

In chronic jaw pain, the nervous system no longer treats clenching as a short-term response. It treats it as an ongoing strategy for threat management. The jaw becomes what can be thought of as a biological cast. Instead of rigid material, the cast is made of constant low-level muscle contraction that never fully releases.

This guarding is meant to protect the joint and surrounding tissues, but it carries a cost. Continuous muscle activity reduces circulation, limits oxygen delivery, and accelerates fatigue. Metabolic byproducts accumulate, increasing chemical irritation in the muscle tissue.

That irritation feeds additional pain signals back into the nervous system, reinforcing the belief that danger is still present. As this cycle continues, the alarm system becomes sensitized. The brain starts responding not only to clear threats, but also to neutral or benign input. Light tooth contact, focused concentration, emotional stress, poor sleep, or even stillness can provoke more guarding.

The threshold for activation remains low, and the system stays locked in high alert. This is why chronic jaw pain often feels unpredictable and hard to calm. The nervous system is no longer asking, "Is this dangerous?" It is assuming that it is.

Until that assumption changes, clenching remains the default posture. Relief requires more than reducing pain intensity. It requires changing how safety is signaled to the nervous system itself.

Safety Signals Versus Threat Signals

To interrupt protective jaw tension, your nervous system must receive signals that outweigh its perception of danger. Threat signals increase vigilance and bracing. Safety signals do the opposite. They inhibit the splinting reflex at a brainstem level and allow muscle tone to downshift without effort.[5,10]

Safety signals work because they compete with pain and threat input rather than confronting it. Gentle vibration, warmth, slow nasal breathing with extended exhalation, and stable tongue posture all communicate safety without demanding performance.

They do not require focus, control, or willpower. Instead, they provide information that the nervous system can accept while staying regulated. This distinction matters.

Many relaxation strategies fail in pain states because they increase vigilance. Trying to force the jaw to relax can feel like work, which the nervous system interprets as more demand. Safety signals succeed because they reduce demand.

This is why neutral biofeedback tools such as ClenchAlert can be effective when pain is present. The vibration is not corrective or punitive. It does not tell the nervous system it is doing something wrong. It simply provides a neutral cue that brings clenching into awareness without triggering further guarding.[7]

Because the signal is informational rather than threatening, it bypasses the alarm response. That allows conscious recalibration to occur while the system remains calm, making change possible without adding more tension.

Practical Ways to Interrupt the Pain–Tension Loop

The most effective strategies address mechanical, neural, and chemical contributors simultaneously.

Neutral awareness interrupts. When a clench is detected, drop the jaw slightly and introduce gentle movement. Small side-to-side motion can help reawaken the sensory map without force.

Respiratory safety cues lengthen the exhale. Vocalized sighs and humming stimulate vagal pathways that actively inhibit jaw motor output.[10,11]

Thermal regulation warmth increases blood flow and reduces muscle viscosity. Brief cooling afterward can dampen nerve excitability. Alternating the two can disrupt static pain signaling.[12]

Postural unloading lifting the sternum and stacking the head over the shoulders reduces the mechanical demand on the jaw to act as an anchor. Consistent neutral posture lips together, teeth apart, tongue resting on the palate creates a physical configuration that is incompatible with sustained clenching.

The Timeline for Change

Protective tension is learned. It is reinforced synaptically. It fades the same way. This is the most important timeline shift to understand because it removes the false expectation that you should be able to think your way out of a body-level reflex.

If your jaw has been bracing for months or years, it has become part of your nervous system's default strategy for stability. The brain has practiced this pattern thousands of times. It has built speed, efficiency, and automaticity. That is why change is not a single decision. It is a process of retraining.

Progress is measured in consistency, not intensity. Most people instinctively try to override clenching with force. They try to "hold the jaw open," stretch aggressively, or command themselves to relax. That often backfires because effort can sound like urgency to the brain, and urgency reads as threat.

The nervous system does not change because you apply more pressure. It changes because you apply the right signal, repeatedly, in a calm tone. Each neutral interruption is a corrective signal. It is a moment where you teach your system: this is not danger, this is just pressure, and I can respond without bracing.

Over time, the nervous system updates its threat model. That phrase matters. Your brain is running an internal prediction all day long: Do I need protection right now. If the answer is yes, muscle tone rises. The jaw tightens.

Breathing gets shallow. Focus narrows. You do not choose this consciously. It is an automatic output of a nervous system trying to keep you safe. Every time you notice tension and respond with a

195

skillful reset, you deliver new evidence. You prove that the situation can be met with awareness rather than armor. You prove that you can stay functional without clenching. That evidence accumulates.

The goal is not to eliminate pain immediately. The goal is to convince the brain that the jaw no longer needs a splint. Pain often triggers protection. Protection increases tone. Increased tone increases pain. If you only chase pain relief, you may accidentally keep feeding the loop by treating every sensation as an emergency.

The more effective approach is quieter and more precise. You aim to reduce the need for guarding. You lower the background level of threat in the body through repeated safe experiences: softening the tongue, lengthening the exhale, decompressing posture, reducing the intensity of focus-bracing, and using neutral cues that interrupt clenching without adding alarm.

This is why small, repeated wins matter more than dramatic interventions. The nervous system trusts pattern. It trusts repetition. If you give it one long session of perfect relaxation and then return to hours of bracing, the brain will keep its old conclusion. If you give it dozens of brief moments of safe interruption across the day, the brain begins to revise its baseline. The jaw starts to loosen sooner. The clenches become lighter. Recovery becomes faster. You may still clench, but you will not stay clenched.

When safety becomes more convincing than threat, the guard finally comes down. That is the real marker of progress. Not a flawless day. A shorter clench. A faster release. A softer baseline. A growing confidence that your body can handle pressure without turning your jaw into a shield.

References

Pain–Motor Adaptation, Guarding, and the Pain–Spasm–Pain Cycle

1. Lund JP, Donga R, Widmer CG, Stohler CS. The pain-adaptation model: a discussion of the relationship between chronic musculoskeletal pain and motor activity. Can J Physiol Pharmacol. 1991;69(5):683-694.

2. Peck CC, Murray GM, Gerzina TM. How does pain affect jaw muscle activity? The integrated pain adaptation model. Aust Dent J. 2008;53(3):201-207. doi:10.1111/j.1834-7819.2008.00050.x

Central Sensitization and Chronic Orofacial Pain Amplification

3. Woolf CJ. Central sensitization: implications for the diagnosis and treatment of pain. Pain. 2011;152(3 Suppl):S2-S15. doi:10.1016/j.pain.2010.09.030

4. Nijs J, Lahousse A, Kapreli E, et al. Nociplastic pain criteria or recognition of central sensitization? Clinical reasoning in chronic pain. J Clin Med. 2021;10(7):1419. doi:10.3390/jcm10071419

Sympathetic Arousal, Stress Chemistry, and Pain-Tension Coupling

5. Melzack R. Pain and the neuromatrix in the brain. J Dent Educ. 2001;65(12):1378-1382.

6.   Hannibal KE, Bishop MD. Chronic stress, cortisol dysfunction, and pain: a psychoneuroendocrine rationale for stress management in pain rehabilitation. Phys Ther. 2014;94(12):1816-1825. doi:10.2522/ptj.20130597

Biofeedback and Operant Learning for Bruxism-Related Behaviors (Mechanism-Level Support)

7.   Vieira MdA, Oliveira-Souza AISd, Hahn G, Bähr L, Armijo-Olivo S, Ferreira APdL. Effectiveness of biofeedback in individuals with awake bruxism compared to other types of treatment: a systematic review. Int J Environ Res Public Health. 2023;20(2):1558. doi:10.3390/ijerph20021558

8.   Lobbezoo F, Ahlberg J, Glaros AG, et al. Bruxism defined and graded: an international consensus. J Oral Rehabil. 2013;40(1):2-4. doi:10.1111/joor.12011

9.   Raphael KG, Janal MN, Sirois DA, et al. Effect of contingent electrical stimulation on masticatory muscle activity and pain in patients with a myofascial temporomandibular disorder and sleep bruxism. J Orofac Pain.2013;27(1):21-32. PubMed

Safety-Cue Physiology (Breathing/Vibration/Warmth) as Downshifting Inputs

10. Lehrer PM, Gevirtz R. Heart rate variability biofeedback: how and why does it work? Front Psychol. 2014;5:756. doi:10.3389/fpsyg.2014.00756

11. Weitzberg E, Lundberg JO. Humming greatly increases nasal nitric oxide. Am J Respir Crit Care Med.2002;166(2):144-145. doi:10.1164/rccm.200202-138BC

12. Nadler SF, Steiner DJ, Erasala GN, et al. Continuous low-level heatwrap therapy provides more efficacy than ibuprofen and acetaminophen for acute low back pain. Spine (Phila Pa 1976). 2002;27(10):1012-1017. doi:10.1097/00007632-200205150-00008

Chapter 13: Emotion, Control, and Holding On

The Emotional Patterns Behind Clenching

Jaw clenching is not only a mechanical habit or a generic "stress response." For many people, it functions as an emotional strategy.[2,3] When feelings are intense, complicated, or hard to express, the nervous system often searches for a place to contain that energy.

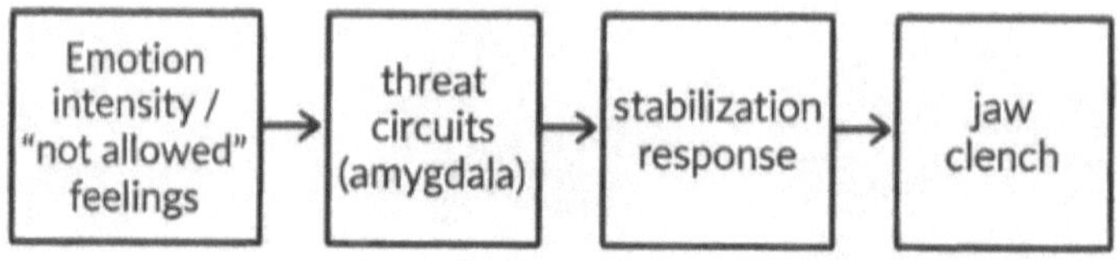

The jaw is a common storage site because it is always available, socially hidden, and easy to tighten without drawing attention. You can brace your jaw in a meeting, in traffic, during conflict, or while trying to stay composed, and no one will notice.

Clenching can serve several emotional purposes at once. It can signal self-control when you feel overwhelmed. It can create a sense of readiness when you feel uncertain. It can act like a lid on anger, grief, fear, or disappointment when those emotions do not feel "allowed."

Over time, the nervous system learns that tightening the jaw is a reliable way to prevent visible reaction.[2] The problem is that what begins as short-term containment can become a long-term pattern.[2]

The jaw starts to brace not only during stress, but during concentration, decision-making, and even rest.

Certain emotional styles make this more likely. Perfectionism often creates a constant background pressure, a belief that mistakes are costly and vigilance is necessary.[8] Suppressed anger can keep the body in a quiet state of readiness, as if you are holding back words, boundaries, or reactions. Emotional control, especially in people who have learned to be the "steady one," can train the nervous system to manage feelings through tension instead of expression.

This is why compassion is not optional in jaw work.[7,8] If your nervous system believes emotions are dangerous, it will keep clenching to contain them. Criticism and force tend to increase guarding. Compassion, in contrast, signals safety. It lowers threat, reduces internal conflict, and makes release biologically possible.

Change is not about trying harder. It is about creating enough safety that your body no longer needs to brace to cope.

Why Emotions Live in the Jaw

The jaw sits at the intersection of communication, power, and restraint. You use it to speak and eat, but also to bite, defend, and hold back. Because of that dual role, the jaw often becomes the body's "braking system" when emotion feels risky to express.

When you cannot say what you mean, show irritation, set a boundary, or admit fear, the nervous system still has to do something with the energy. One common solution is tension.

Neurologically, emotional threat can activate the same survival circuits as physical threat. The amygdala flags danger, even if the danger is internal and social, such as fear of failure, conflict avoidance, shame, or the pressure to stay composed.

That alarm signal engages the brainstem and increases baseline muscle tone. The jaw can brace as part of a broader stabilization response that includes facial tension, tongue rigidity, and neck and shoulder tightening.

It is not a conscious decision. It is a protective posture.

Over time, this turns into a learned pattern.[2,4] The jaw tightens during hard conversations, decision-making, performance pressure, or even quiet concentration. Eventually, the tension can persist even when nothing is happening externally.[2,5]

The jaw becomes a container for emotional labor, holding what you do not feel safe to express, and doing it so consistently that clenching starts to feel normal.

Perfectionism and Jaw Clenching

Perfectionism is one of the most reliable emotional drivers of chronic jaw clenching. It is not simply the desire to do well. It is a nervous-system state built on constant self-monitoring and fear of error.

When your brain is scanning for what could go wrong, your body stays on alert. That vigilance requires control, and control often shows up physically as bracing. The jaw becomes a natural place for that bracing. Clenching can feel like "holding effort in place," as if tension helps you stay sharp, steady, or prepared.

Perfectionistic thinking often carries implicit commands to tighten, such as: I must not mess this up. I need to keep it together. I can't relax yet. Even if those thoughts are quiet or automatic, the body responds as if there is something at stake.

Because clenching is often unconscious, many people only notice it after discomfort appears. Then perfectionism adds a second problem: judgment. You catch yourself clenching and immediately label it a failure, another thing you should have fixed.[6,8]

That self-criticism activates the threat system again, increasing muscle tone and making bracing more likely.[8] This is why "trying harder" rarely works. The goal is not perfect relaxation. The goal is earlier awareness and a calmer response when you notice tension.

When you treat clenching as information rather than a mistake, you reduce threat signals and make release physiologically possible.

Suppressed Anger and Contained Emotion

Anger is one of the most frequently suppressed emotions in people who live with chronic jaw tension. Anger carries strong motor energy. It prepares the body to speak plainly, set a boundary, push back, or defend. When that impulse feels unsafe, inappropriate, or "not allowed," the nervous system still has to manage the activation. A common strategy is to redirect it inward and tighten the muscles that help you hold back.

The jaw is well suited for this role. It is involved in biting and speaking, so it becomes a natural control point when you are inhibiting reaction. The jaw can function like a lock, keeping emotion contained even while your system is mobilized underneath.

This often happens in people who have learned internal rules such as: Don't say that. Don't react. Stay calm. Be professional. Each rule requires inhibition, and inhibition has a physical footprint. The jaw clenches to enforce restraint.

Clenching allows anger to exist without outward expression.[4,5] In the moment, it can create the feeling that you are in control. But the cost is constant muscular effort, reduced recovery, and a nervous system that stays activated longer than it needs to.

Over time, your brain begins to pair emotional containment with physical bracing.[2,5] The pattern becomes automatic.[1,2] You may not

203

feel "angry," but your jaw is still holding the posture of anger, long after the moment has passed.

Why Control Feels Safer Than Release

For many people, holding tension feels safer than letting it go.[7,8] Control creates predictability. It keeps you organized, composed, and ready. Release, by contrast, can feel uncertain. If your nervous system equates "softening" with vulnerability, then letting go does not register as relief. It registers as risk, like losing stability, losing composure, or even losing a familiar sense of who you are.

This is why the body may maintain jaw tension long after the original stressor has passed. The nervous system is not tracking the calendar. It is tracking safety. If tension has become your default way of staying steady, it will persist even in quiet moments, because the system has learned that bracing equals protection.

It also explains why forcing relaxation often backfires. Trying to relax by effort is still a form of control. It adds pressure, increases monitoring, and can make you more aware of every sensation in the jaw. Instead of signaling safety, the nervous system hears another demand: Fix this. Get it right. Try harder. That demand can raise vigilance and increase muscle tone.

True release is not something you impose. It is something your nervous system allows when it has evidence that softening is safe. That evidence often comes from small, repeatable safety cues: slower exhalation, gentle jaw drops, warm compresses, stable tongue posture, or neutral biofeedback that helps you notice tension early without triggering self-criticism. Over time, those cues retrain the system to downshift.

Compassion as a Neurobiological Intervention

Compassion is not merely a mindset. It is a physiological signal that changes how your nervous system interprets what is happening in your body. When you notice clenching and respond with judgment, you add threat to an already activated system.[8]

The brain reads criticism as danger, the amygdala stays engaged, and baseline muscle tone remains elevated. In that state, your body is more likely to brace again, not less.

When you respond with understanding, the signal is different. You are telling your nervous system, "This is not an emergency."[6,7] That reduces perceived threat and makes downshifting possible. Validation does not mean you like the symptom or want it to continue. It means you recognize the clench as information, not a personal failure. That distinction matters because the nervous system cannot release what it still believes it must defend against.

Compassion also improves awareness. If you expect yourself to be perfect, you will avoid noticing tension because noticing it feels like bad news. If you can observe tension without punishment, you can detect it earlier, when it is easier to interrupt. Earlier awareness reduces intensity, reduces duration, and prevents the escalation into full protective bracing.

This is where compassion becomes a mechanism for change, not a soft concept. It lowers threat chemistry, reduces guarding, and creates the internal conditions needed for the jaw to soften. In practical terms, compassion is a stability cue. It tells your brain that you can feel discomfort, emotion, or stress without having to clamp down to survive it.

The Compassionate Scan

A CBT-Based Somatic Release

205

A somatic release is a brief, body-based reset that helps your nervous system let go of protective tension. It is not a dramatic "letting go" moment and it is not a forceful relaxation technique. A somatic release is simply the practice of noticing what your body is doing, naming it without judgment, and giving it a small, safe cue to soften.

The goal is not to make tension disappear on command. The goal is to interrupt the automatic pattern before it escalates into pain, fatigue, or a full clench.

From a CBT perspective, this matters because jaw clenching is often maintained by a habit loop: a trigger, an automatic response, and a short-term sense of control or stability. The body learns that bracing feels protective, even when it causes problems later. Somatic release works by changing the middle of that loop.

Instead of responding to stress or emotion with tightening, you practice a new response that your nervous system can tolerate. Over time, that new response becomes more available and more automatic.

The Compassionate Scan is a structured way to do this. You briefly scan for common holding points, especially in the jaw, tongue, face, neck, and shoulders. You do not "hunt" for problems.

Step-by-step micro practice card

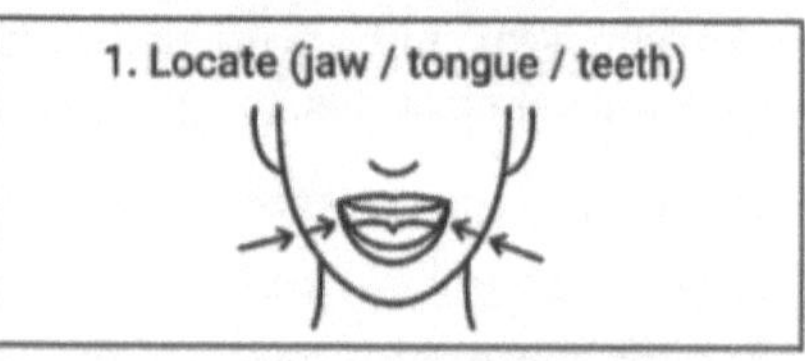

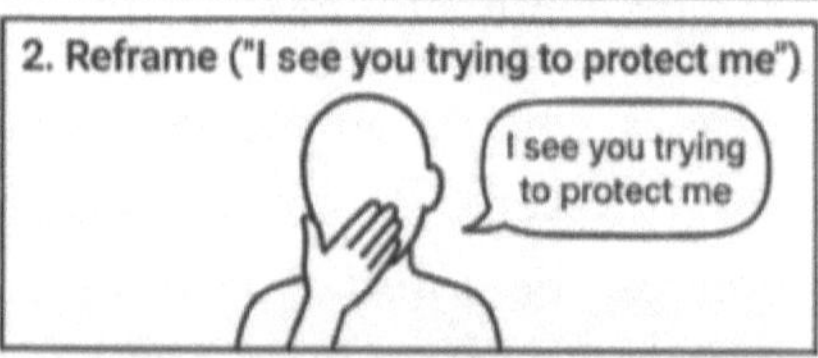

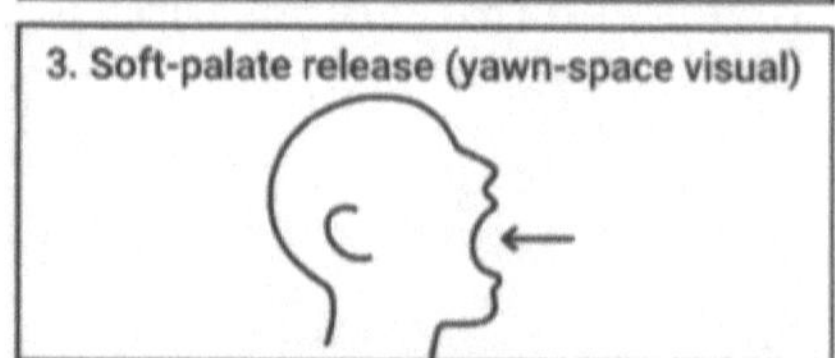

Normalizes recurrence and reframes dips as part of growth

You observe. Then you apply a gentle release cue, paired with a calm interpretation: nothing is wrong, and you are safe to soften. This combination, awareness plus compassion, is what retrains the system. It is how you teach your body that release is not loss of control. It is a safer form of control.

Step 1: Physical localization

Close your eyes and take a breath. Do not try to change anything. Notice your jaw as it is. Observe the action tendency. Are your teeth touching. Is your tongue pressing upward. Is your jaw rigid or held.

Ask a simple CBT-style question: If this clench were a word, what would it be. Common answers include wait, no, hold, push, quiet.

Step 2: The compassionate reframe

Instead of criticizing the tension, acknowledge its role. Silently say: I see you trying to protect me. I see you holding the stress so I do not have to feel it all at once. Thank you for trying to keep me safe. This reframing deactivates the amygdala. When the threat center quiets, the protective splinting reflex loses its fuel.

Step 3: The soft-palate release

Rather than forcing the jaw open, soften the structures behind it. Imagine the space between your back molars widening. Visualize the soft palate lifting slightly, as if beginning a gentle yawn.

Let the tongue rest heavily in the floor of the mouth for ten seconds, like a tired muscle that no longer needs to work. This sensory shift interrupts the holding pattern and allows the jaw muscles to lengthen naturally.

Using Biofeedback as a Compassion Cue

If you use ClenchAlert, the most important factor is not the vibration itself. It is how you interpret the vibration in the moment. In a CBT practice, biofeedback is not a correction tool. It is a cue for awareness and a prompt for a new response.[9,10] When the vibration is framed as a mistake, it can feed perfectionism.

You notice the signal and immediately think, "I failed again," or "I should be past this." That interpretation activates the threat system, increases muscle tone, and makes bracing more likely. The device becomes associated with pressure, and the nervous system learns to stay on guard.

Used differently, the same vibration can retrain safety. When you treat the cue as neutral information, it becomes a moment of permission: "My body is trying to protect me. I can respond with softness." That shift matters because the nervous system does not change through willpower alone. It changes when it receives repeated evidence that releasing tension is safe. In practical terms, biofeedback supports CBT by reducing the burden of constant self-monitoring.

You do not have to catch every clench through effort. The cue helps you notice earlier, when the tension is still light and easier to interrupt. Your job is simple: pause, exhale slowly, let the tongue rest, allow the jaw to separate, and move on without self-criticism. Over time, this pairing, cue plus compassionate response, weakens the clench habit loop and builds a new default: awareness without alarm, and release without struggle.

When the vibration occurs:

Old Pattern	Compassionate Pattern
I am doing it again. I failed.	My body is bracing. It thinks I am under pressure.
Force the jaw open.	Soften the eyes and tongue.
Tension plus frustration.	Awareness plus safety.

The vibration is not an alarm. It is information. When treated neutrally, it becomes a bridge between unconscious reflex and conscious choice.

Reference

Bruxism, stress physiology, and psychosocial drivers

1. Lobbezoo F, Ahlberg J, Raphael KG, et al. International consensus on the assessment of bruxism: Report of a work in progress. J Oral Rehabil. 2018;45(11):837-844. doi:10.1111/joor.12663

2. Manfredini D, Lobbezoo F. Role of psychosocial factors in the etiology of bruxism. J Orofac Pain.2009;23(2):153-166.

3. Emodi-Perlman A, Eli I, Smardz J, et al. Temporomandibular disorders and bruxism outbreak as a possible factor of orofacial pain worsening during the COVID-19 pandemic—concomitant research in two countries. J Clin Med. 2020;9(10):3250. doi:10.3390/jcm9103250

Emotion regulation, anger, control styles, and orofacial pain/TMD

4. Wieckiewicz M, Boening K, Wiland P, Shiau YY, Paradowska-Stolarz A. Reported concepts for the treatment modalities and pain management of temporomandibular disorders. J Headache Pain. 2015;16:106. doi:10.1186/s10194-015-0586-5

5. Ohrbach R, Dworkin SF. The evolution of TMD diagnosis: Past, present, future. J Dent Res. 2016;95(10):1093-1101. doi:10.1177/0022034516653922

Self-criticism/perfectionism mechanisms, threat appraisal, and self-compassion as a downshifting signal

6. Neff KD. Self-compassion: An alternative conceptualization of a healthy attitude toward oneself. Self Identity.2003;2(2):85-101. doi:10.1080/15298860309032

7. Leaviss J, Uttley L. Psychotherapeutic benefits of compassion-focused therapy: An early systematic review. Psychol Med. 2015;45(5):927-945. doi:10.1017/S0033291714002141

8. Longe O, Maratos FA, Gilbert P, Evans G, Volker F, Rockliff H, Rippon G. Having a word with yourself: Neural correlates of self-criticism and self-reassurance. Neuroimage. 2010;49(2):1849-1856. doi:10.1016/j.neuroimage.2009.09.019

Biofeedback and operant learning

9. Jadidi F, Castrillon EE, Svensson P. Effect of contingent electrical stimulation on jaw muscle activity during sleep: A randomized controlled trial. J Oral Rehabil. 2013;40(3):231-239. doi:10.1111/joor.12031

10. Ohara H, Tsukiyama Y, Ogawa T, Koyano K. Effects of vibratory feedback stimuli through an oral appliance on sleep bruxism: A randomized controlled trial. Sleep Breath. 2022;26(4):1565-1573. doi:10.1007/s11325-021-02463-3

Part V: Exchange: Sustaining Change

Transform short-term awareness into a lasting relationship with your body

Meet Lena.

Lena was six weeks into her BRUX practice, and the change felt real. Her jaw stayed softer through the day. Her mornings were lighter. The familiar ache that used to greet her at breakfast had faded into the background. Even her ClenchAlert had become quiet. The buzzing that once interrupted her often was now rare, almost a confirmation that her baseline was shifting.

Then life compressed.

A week arrived that would have challenged anyone's regulation. Deadlines stacked up. One of the kids got sick, then the other. Sleep became fragmented, with late-night wakeups and early mornings. Meals were rushed. Hydration slipped. Her nervous system was running on borrowed capacity, and by the time Thursday hit, she noticed something she hadn't felt in weeks: the ClenchAlert buzzing again.

Her first thought was immediate and familiar: I've failed. For a moment, she wanted to rip the device out, frustrated with herself and tired of the work. But instead of reacting, she paused. She noticed the urge to judge, and she recognized what it meant: her system was overloaded, not broken. She took a slow breath, let her shoulders drop, and softened her jaw on the exhale. Then she did something small that changed everything. She smiled, almost gently, and whispered, "Hello again." It was not denial. It was orientation. That simple phrase shifted her from threat to curiosity. It reminded her that clenching is a protective reflex that reappears when load exceeds capacity

. The buzzing was not a verdict. It was information.

That evening, Lena opened her journal and wrote one sentence that clarified the difference between relapse and learning: "I realized I'm not starting over. I'm reinforcing what I've learned." That was her turning point. She stopped treating recurrence as failure and started treating it as practice under pressure.

The week did not erase her progress. It revealed the edges of her current capacity and gave her a clear target for adjustment: more micro-resets, earlier decompression, and a little more compassion during high-demand seasons.

From that point forward, the return of symptoms no longer meant she was back at zero. It meant she had an opportunity to rehearse the new skill in the exact conditions that used to trigger the old pattern. Her relapse became rehearsal, and rehearsal became stability.

Chapter 14: From Habit to Harmony

Reframing Relapse as Information and Replacing Self Criticism with Curiosity and Skillful Adjustment

Progress with clenching almost never follows a straight, upward line.[5] You may have several calm weeks, then one high-demand day lands, your shoulders rise, your breath shortens, and your jaw tightens before you even notice. When that happens, it can feel discouraging, especially if your nervous system is wired for perfectionism and expects that once you improve, the improvement should hold permanently. This chapter reframes "relapse" as feedback rather than failure. A return of clenching is not a moral verdict and it is not proof that nothing is working.[5,8,9] It is a data point. It tells you something

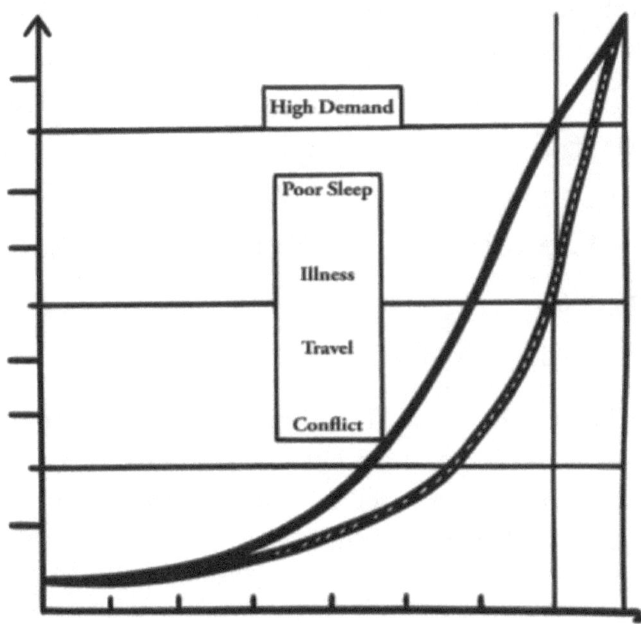

specific about load, capacity, and your body's protective patterning in that moment. Stress, fatigue, sensory overload, conflict, long screen time, dehydration, pain, or poor sleep can all narrow your margin.[6,7,11]

When the margin narrows, the nervous system defaults to what it has practiced most: bracing.[2,3,6] When you treat recurrence as information, your strategy changes. You stop arguing with your physiology and you start training it. Instead of "What is wrong with me?" the question becomes "What shifted?" What was different about the day, the environment, the demands, or the timing?

Did you miss your usual cues? Did you skip the small resets that keep the system regulated? Did you hold your breath while concentrating? Did your tongue posture disappear when you got rushed?

Curiosity replaces self-criticism, and curiosity creates options. From there, you can make a skillful adjustment: shorten your work sprints, add a 30-second jaw check-in, re-anchor breath, soften the tongue, drop the shoulders, or use a neutral prompt such as biofeedback to catch the pattern earlier.

Harmony is not never clenching. Harmony is noticing sooner, recovering faster, and adjusting without self-attack.

Why Clenching Can Return Even After Progress

The Neurological Echo.

Your brain is designed for efficiency, not perfection.[2,3] When you practice relaxation and jaw release, you build new neural pathways that support a calmer baseline. However, those new pathways do not erase the old clenching circuit.[4,5]

The original pattern remains stored in the nervous system, dormant rather than deleted. It exists because, at one time, it worked. It helped you concentrate, contain emotion, or stabilize under pressure.

When demand suddenly rises and regulation resources dip, the brain often reaches for the most familiar and well-rehearsed strategy.[2,3,7] This is not regression. It is the nervous system choosing speed over novelty.[2,3,7]

The return of clenching does not mean the new habit failed. It means the older habit still has a strong signal because it was practiced for years. Understanding this removes moral judgment from the experience. You are not "backsliding." You are witnessing the nervous system doing what it evolved to do: protect efficiently when conditions tighten.

When Load Exceeds Capacity

Relapse most often appears during periods of heightened demand.[5,6] Deadlines, conflict, travel, illness, pain, dehydration, poor sleep, or major emotional transitions all increase nervous system load. The pattern is not random, and it is not a personal flaw.

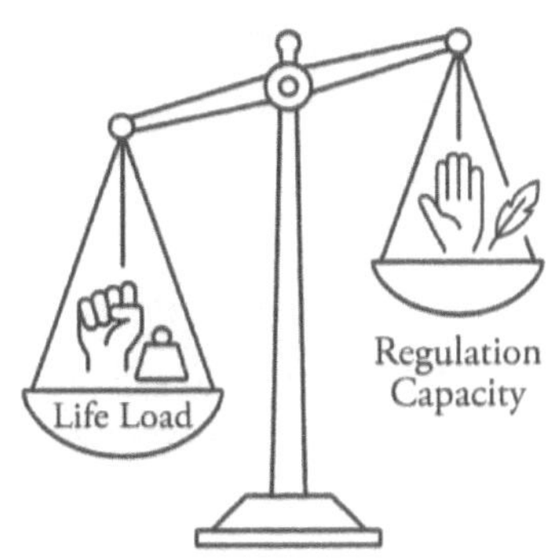

When load > capacity → brace response

The common factor is that total demand rises faster than available regulatory capacity.[6,7] In cognitive behavioral terms, your trigger threshold is not fixed. It shifts based on internal state. When you are rested, nourished, supported, and emotionally regulated, the system can absorb stress without bracing. When those supports erode, even familiar stressors can push you past threshold.

Seen this way, clenching becomes a signal rather than a failure. It tells you that capacity is temporarily reduced or load has quietly accumulated. This perspective invites problem-solving instead of self-criticism.

You can respond by reducing inputs, increasing recovery, or adding supports, rather than trying to force control over a nervous system that is already stretched.

Protect First, Explain Later

Clenching is a rapid bracing response driven by subcortical circuitry. It often activates before conscious awareness, especially during sustained concentration, emotional restraint, or high cognitive demand. The brain's priority is protection, not explanation.

It stabilizes first and makes sense of the action later, if at all. Because of this timing, the goal is not to eliminate every clench in real time. That expectation creates frustration and vigilance, which can increase tension. The more effective goal is to shorten the loop. Faster detection. Quicker release. Cleaner recovery.

When a clench becomes brief and noticeable rather than prolonged and unconscious, it shifts from a costly pattern to a useful data point. Tools such as deliberate check-ins, posture resets, breath cues, or neutral biofeedback can support this process without adding pressure. Over time, the nervous system learns that release is available sooner, and the protective response no longer needs to persist.

The Cost of Self Criticism

Self-criticism is not neutral. Your nervous system often reads it as a threat. When you catch yourself clenching and think, "I'm doing it again. This is ridiculous. I'll never change," your brain does not file that as helpful motivation. It registers it as an internal attack. That appraisal increases arousal, activates stress circuitry, and raises baseline muscle tone. In other words, the exact physiology you are trying to reduce gets reinforced.

This creates a predictable paradox: the shame about clenching can increase the clenching. Relapse then becomes a two-part problem. First, the jaw tightens in response to load. Second, the self-judgment adds a fresh layer of threat, which tells the body to brace even more. The system is not being stubborn.

It is following its core job description: protect you when it senses danger. If recurrence is met with force, frustration, or punishment, the nervous system receives a clear signal that conditions are unsafe. When conditions feel unsafe, the body does not learn release. It rehearses protection. A more effective response is to treat the moment as data: notice, soften, reset, and adjust without self-attack.

Why Curiosity Works Better Than Judgment

Curiosity works because it changes your state before it changes your strategy. When you become curious, the nervous system shifts out of urgency. Attention widens. Breathing often slows. The body gets a subtle signal that it can afford to observe rather than brace.

You cannot stay deeply curious and deeply panicked at the same time because the two states compete for the same bandwidth. Judgment narrows attention and raises threat. Curiosity does the opposite.

It opens a problem-solving channel. When you ask, "What changed?" instead of "What is wrong with me?" you move from self-attack to investigation.

That single shift lowers protective tone and makes it easier to notice the actual variables: fatigue, deadlines, sensory overload, conflict, screen time, dehydration, pain, or emotional suppression. Curiosity is not permissive, and it is not a soft excuse. It is a functional stance that supports regulation and skill building.

It helps you identify patterns without adding stress to the system. It also produces better decisions because it keeps you oriented to cause and effect rather than identity and blame. In practice, curiosity turns recurrence into useful information. You can adjust load, increase recovery, and refine your reset tools. Over time, the jaw becomes a signal you can respond to, not a verdict you have to fear.

Relapse as a Data Point

When clenching returns, treat it as information rather than failure. In most cases, it points to one of four load categories that temporarily push your nervous system past threshold. The goal is not to diagnose yourself.

The goal is to identify which type of load increased so you can make a practical adjustment. Ask: What was different today? What demand rose, what support dropped, and what did my body do to compensate?

Once you name the category, you can respond with the right tool, not more effort. Clenching becomes a signal that guides your next step, not a verdict about your progress.

Cognitive Load

Cognitive load is the mental strain of sustained thinking and rapid task switching. Long work blocks, intense focus, problem-solving under time pressure, and high-stakes communication can all drive unconscious bracing. You may hold your breath, lift your shoulders, or push your tongue down while concentrating. The jaw then tightens as part of a full-body "get it done" pattern.

The adjustment is usually structural and behavioral: shorten focus sprints, add brief check-ins, relax the tongue, exhale fully, and reset posture before the tension accumulates.

Emotional Load

Emotional load increases when you are managing feelings that are intense, complex, or socially constrained. Perfectionism, suppressed anger, resentment, conflict avoidance, grief, and uncertainty often show up as jaw tension because the mouth is a natural "containment" zone.

You may clench to stay composed, to avoid saying something, or to keep moving through discomfort. The adjustment is not forcing relaxation. It is creating safer expression and regulation: name the emotion, soften the face, unclench on the exhale, and choose a response that reduces internal holding.

Structural Load

Structural load is the mechanical strain that builds when your body is positioned for bracing. Forward head posture, screen height, jaw position, shoulder tension, breath holding, and sleep posture can all increase baseline jaw muscle tone. When your head drifts forward, the neck and jaw often co-contract for stability. The jaw then tightens as a stabilizer, not as a choice. The adjustment is environmental and

221

ergonomic: raise screens, stack head over ribs, drop shoulders, keep lips together with the tongue resting up, and build frequent micro-resets.

Chemical Load

Chemical load refers to internal physiology that raises irritability and reduces recovery capacity. Poor sleep rhythm, dehydration, caffeine timing, under fueling, hormone shifts, pain sensitivity, and inflammation can all lower your threshold and amplify muscle reactivity.

On those days, even minor stress can trigger clenching because the system is already "hot." The adjustment is supportive, not disciplinary: stabilize sleep timing, hydrate earlier, time caffeine strategically, eat consistently, and reduce late-day stimulation. When the internal terrain improves, the jaw often follows. Relapse becomes useful the moment it is categorized.

The Harmony Matrix

Shifting Your Response in Real Time:

Event	Habit Response (Self Criticism)	Harmony Response (Curiosity)
Clenching returns	"All that work is wasted."	"Interesting. My system is overloaded. What changed?"
Pain appears	"Something is wrong with me."	"Pain is a signal. I need to decompress and soften inputs."
Biofeedback cue	"Stop it. Why am I doing this?"	"Thank you. This is my early warning signal."

Event	Habit Response (Self Criticism)	Harmony Response (Curiosity)
Setback day	"I need more willpower."	"I need a better adjustment. Smaller resets, sooner."

Harmony is not an emotional pep talk. It is a better operating system.

The Curiosity Audit

A 10-Second Relapse Check-In

When you catch clenching, run this quick audit. Do not overthink it. Pick one answer and pivot.

1. What was my mental tab? What was I trying to solve, control, or prevent?

2. Where is my breath? Was I holding it? Was it shallow? Was I in upper chest breathing?

3. What is my posture? Was my head forward? Was my sternum collapsed? Was I leaning on one elbow?

4. What is my chemical state? Am I dehydrated? Underfueled? Overcaffeinated? Sleep deprived?

This audit turns relapse into a map.

Skillful Adjustment

Replace Trying Harder with Adjusting Better

Once you identify the likely driver, choose a single, precise adjustment. If the driver is breath holding Start with a long, slow exhale. Let the exhale be slightly longer than the inhale to signal

223

"downshift" to the nervous system. As you exhale, allow the tongue to rest heavy and wide, with the tip lightly behind the upper front teeth. Keep your lips together and let your teeth separate without forcing the jaw open. Drop the shoulders and unclench the hands as well, because the jaw often mirrors global bracing.

Repeat for three breaths.

The objective is not perfect calm. It is to interrupt the breath-hold pattern early and restore airflow, which reduces jaw tone.

If the driver is posture

Make a small, mechanical reset. Gently lift the sternum, then lengthen the back of the neck as if creating space between the ears and shoulders.

Re-stack the head over the shoulders rather than craning toward the screen. Let the jaw hang lightly, keeping lips together while teeth remain apart. Check "freeway space," the natural gap between upper and lower teeth at rest.

If you are at a desk, raise the screen and bring the work closer to you, not your face closer to the work. A posture reset works best when it is small, frequent, and non-dramatic.

If the driver is cognitive load

Reduce intensity before pain forces you to. Shorten the next work block and build a micro-reset into transitions, not only into breaks. For example, every time you open a new tab, send an email, or start a meeting, do a 10-second check: exhale, tongue up, lips together, teeth apart, shoulders down. This keeps the nervous system from accumulating silent tension.

Avoid waiting for the jaw to "scream" because by then the system is already in protective mode. The point is proactive regulation. Small resets practiced early create more change than big resets practiced late. If the driver is emotional restraint.

Meet the moment with compassionate accuracy rather than command-and-control. Use a simple internal statement: "My body is bracing. It believes I need protection."

That framing reduces shame and lowers threat, which makes release more possible. Then soften the face on the exhale, unclench the tongue, and allow the jaw to separate slightly. If you can, name the emotion you are holding, even quietly: anger, fear, grief, pressure, uncertainty. Emotional restraint often recruits the jaw to "hold it together." Your goal is to give the nervous system a safer option than bracing, not to force calm.

If the driver is dehydration or fatigue:

Treat this as a resource problem, not a discipline problem. Hydrate promptly and consider electrolytes if you have been sweating, traveling, or drinking significant caffeine.

Eat something with protein and complex carbohydrate if you are under fueled. Then lower the intensity of the next hour: reduce multitasking, shorten tasks, and avoid high-stakes conversations if you can.

Fatigue reduces your regulation bandwidth, and dehydration increases muscle reactivity, which makes clenching more likely and harder to release. Regulation becomes dramatically easier when the body has basic inputs. The most skillful move is often to support the physiology first, then return to training.

Skillful adjustment is how a nervous system learns safety under pressure.

Using ClenchAlert as a Curiosity Catcher

ClenchAlert is most effective when it is treated as information, not correction.

When the device vibrates:

Note the context
What was I doing or thinking.

Choose one adjustment
Breath, posture, or a quick softening cue.

Acknowledge the win
Noticing is success. The goal is not never clenching. The goal is noticing quickly and recovering efficiently. This transforms the device from a reminder of failure into a guide toward refinement.

The New Definition of Success

Success is not a jaw that never tightens. A healthy nervous system will always respond to challenge, concentration, conflict, excitement, or uncertainty. The goal is not to eliminate response. The goal is to restore flexibility. Success is a jaw that no longer has to stay tight. That distinction matters because chronic clenching is rarely about a single moment of tension. It is about duration.

It is about the jaw becoming the place your body stores pressure when it does not know where else to put it. When you redefine success this way, you stop chasing an unrealistic standard and start building something more durable: a system that can feel stress without turning it into armor. You are building a new response pattern. Under pressure, the old pathway was bracing. Clench, hold, push through. That pattern is not a character flaw. It is a survival strategy that once felt useful. It gave your nervous system a sense of stability, control, and readiness. But over time, it became costly. It raised your baseline muscle tone, amplified pain sensitivity, and taught your body that focus requires force. The new pathway is different. The new pathway meets pressure with awareness instead of bracing.

It meets discomfort with support instead of self attack. It replaces urgency with skill. It replaces shame with information. Each time you notice tension and respond with a small reset, you are not just releasing your jaw. You are teaching your nervous system what safety feels like in real time.

This is why curiosity is essential. Self criticism acts like a threat signal. It tells the brain something is wrong, which increases sympathetic arousal and makes bracing more likely. Curiosity does the opposite. Curiosity keeps you in a regulated state where learning can occur.

When you think, Interesting, my jaw is active right now, you create space between the trigger and the response. That space is where change happens. Over time, the old pathway becomes less compelling. The nervous system still remembers it, but it reaches for it less often. The new pathway becomes more automatic because you have practiced it repeatedly, in ordinary moments, not just during crises. Harmony becomes the default not because life becomes easier, but because your body becomes more responsive.

This is also why relapse deserves a new interpretation. Relapse is not evidence you are back where you started. It is evidence you are learning where you still need support. A return of clenching is a data point. It often means your load exceeded your current capacity, your posture slipped, your breathing became shallow, your sleep was disrupted, or an emotion went unprocessed. The clench is not the failure. The clench is the signal.

The real marker of progress is how quickly you notice, how gently you respond, and how effectively you adjust. When you can catch tension earlier, soften sooner, and recover faster, you are winning. That is the new definition of success.

227

If you want the next chapter to be more practical, I can write a one page Relapse Roadmap that lists the top triggers, the most likely driver category, and the exact skillful adjustment to use in each environment such as desk work, driving, phone calls, and evenings.

References

Bruxism as Behavior, Nervous-System Driven Patterning

1. Lobbezoo F, Ahlberg J, Raphael KG, et al. International consensus on the assessment of bruxism: report of a work in progress. J Oral Rehabil. 2018;45(11):837-844. doi:10.1111/joor.12663

Habit Circuits, Automaticity, and Why Old Patterns Persist

2. Wood W, Rünger D. Psychology of habit. Annu Rev Psychol. 2016;67:289-314. doi:10.1146/annurev-psych-122414-03341

3. Graybiel AM. Habits, rituals, and the evaluative brain. Annu Rev Neurosci. 2008;31:359-387. doi:10.1146/annurev.neuro.29.051605.112851

Learning Theory: Extinction, Relapse, and "Return of an Old Response"

4. Bouton ME. Context, time, and memory retrieval in the interference paradigms of Pavlovian learning. Psychol Bull. 1993;114(1):80-99. doi:10.1037/0033-2909.114.1.80

5. Bouton ME. Why behavior change is difficult to sustain. Prev Med. 2014;68:29-36. doi:10.1016/j.ypmed.2014.06.010

Load, Capacity, and Allostatic Stress Framing

6. McEwen BS. Protective and damaging effects of stress mediators. N Engl J Med. 1998;338(3):171-179. doi:10.1056/NEJM199801153380307

Attention, Cognitive Control, and Fatigue Under Stress

7. Arnsten AFT. Stress signalling pathways that impair prefrontal cortex structure and function. Nat Rev Neurosci.2009;10(6):410-422. doi:10.1038/nrn2648

Self-Criticism, Threat Physiology, and Self-Compassion as a Regulator

8. Gilbert P. The evolution and social dynamics of compassion. Soc Personal Psychol Compass. 2015;9(6):239-254. doi:10.1111/spc3.12176

9. Neff KD. Self-compassion: an alternative conceptualization of a healthy attitude toward oneself. Self Identity.2003;2(2):85-101. doi:10.1080/15298860309032

Curiosity, Mindfulness, and Skillful Observation (State Change Before Strategy Change)

10. Brewer JA. Habit change: a mindfulness-based approach. Curr Opin Psychol. 2019;28:16-20. doi:10.1016/j.copsyc.2018.10.011

Pain/Stress Amplification Loops (Why Emergency-Mode Reactivity Can Entrench Patterns)

11. Wiech K, Tracey I. The influence of negative emotions on pain: behavioral effects and neural mechanisms. Neuroimage. 2009;47(3):987-994. doi:10.1016/j.neuroimage.2009.05.059

12. Schwartz MS, Andrasik F, eds. Biofeedback: A Practitioner's Guide. 4th ed. Guilford Press; 2017.

13. de Albuquerque Vieira R, Oliveira-Souza AIS, Hahn L, Bähr S, Armijo-Olivo S, Ferreira PH. Effectiveness of biofeedback in individuals with awake bruxism compared to other types of treatment: a systematic review. Int J Environ Res Public Health. 2023;20(2):1558. doi:10.3390/ijerph20021558

Chapter 15: Designing Daily Rituals

Lasting jaw relief rarely comes from trying harder to relax in the moment. It comes from building a day that does not require constant self-correction. When your routine is designed to support regulation, tension has fewer chances to accumulate unnoticed. The jaw is not an isolated problem to be managed one clench at a time.

It is a downstream expression of how your nervous system is carrying load across the day.[4,8] This chapter is about the architecture of your routine. It focuses on small, repeatable rituals that reduce baseline arousal and create more consistent neuromuscular

harmony. Think of these rituals as environmental and behavioral supports that keep you closer to your therapeutic "resting state" without needing willpower.

They are not dramatic interventions. They are quiet defaults that make jaw release more likely.[1,2] The shift is subtle but operationally important. You move from sporadic fixes applied after pain appears to rhythmic practices that prevent the build-up in the first place.

Instead of waiting for symptoms to alert you, you install checkpoints that catch early signs of bracing and redirect them. You are not asking yourself to be vigilant all day. You are creating predictable moments when your body is invited to reset.[2,3]

This approach also reduces the emotional cost of change. When your plan depends on remembering to relax, every lapse can feel like failure. When your plan depends on structure, lapses become less frequent and less intense because the day itself carries some of the work.

You are no longer trying to overpower a protective nervous system. You are collaborating with it by giving it regular cues of safety, pacing, and recovery.[5,2] Over time, these small rituals compound. You notice clenching sooner. You recover faster. Your jaw stops being the place where stress collects.

Relief becomes less about heroic effort and more about intelligent design: a day that supports breathing, posture, fuel, and emotional regulation so your nervous system does not need to brace to get you through it.[4,2]

From Effort to Rhythm

Clenching is a reactive behavior. It tends to appear when pressure rises, focus intensifies, emotion is contained, or fatigue narrows your capacity. Because it is reactive and often unconscious, trying to "catch it" with willpower alone becomes exhausting and unreliable.

You may do well for a few hours, then lose track during a call, while driving, or in a stressful conversation. That is not a character flaw. It is how the nervous system works when it is managing load.[5,8] Rituals solve this by reducing the need for moment-to-moment self-monitoring.

A ritual is a repeatable action tied to a predictable cue. It makes regulation easier because it becomes automatic.

Instead of asking your nervous system to remember to relax, you build relaxation into behaviors that already happen without effort: opening your laptop, walking into a meeting, pouring coffee, getting into the car, brushing your teeth.[1,2] This is where habit stacking matters. You attach a brief regulation practice to an existing routine so it rides on the same trigger. For example: after you sit down to work, you exhale slowly and reset tongue posture.

After you send an email, you drop your shoulders and re-check "lips together, teeth apart." After you stand up, you lengthen the back of your neck. Over time, these micro-stacks create rhythm. Regulation stops being an emergency fix and becomes part of how your day runs.[3,2]

The Power of Habit Stacking

Habit stacking is a practical tool from behavioral change science that helps you build new patterns without relying on motivation. It works by attaching a small new behavior to an existing routine that already happens on autopilot. The existing routine becomes the cue, and the new behavior becomes the automatic follow-through.[3,2]

The structure is straightforward: after you complete a familiar habit, you perform a brief jaw reset. Because the first habit is already wired into your day, the second behavior inherits its reliability. You are not asking yourself to remember. You are not negotiating with resistance. You are simply following a sequence that repeats because the cue repeats.[2,3] For jaw health, habit stacking is particularly effective because it creates proactive regulation. Bruxism patterns often build quietly, then announce themselves as pain, headache, or fatigue. Stacks prevent that buildup by clearing tension repeatedly before it becomes entrenched.

A 10-second reset applied ten times a day can be more effective than a long relaxation attempt at the end of the day.[2,4] Examples are simple and flexible: after you open your laptop, exhale and set "lips together, teeth apart." After you send a message, drop your shoulders and let the tongue rest up. After you stand up, re-stack your head over your shoulders. Over time, these micro-resets become rhythm, and your baseline jaw tone often follows.[1,11]

The Morning Practice

Morning is when your nervous system sets its baseline for the day. If you begin the day compressed, guarded, or holding your breath, that protective tone often carries forward for hours. The jaw then becomes an early "holding point" for pressure, even before anything stressful happens. [4,5]

This is why mornings matter. They are less about productivity and more about calibration. The purpose of a morning ritual is simple: establish a lower resting motor tone before demands start arriving. You are teaching your system that safety and steadiness are available first, not only after the day gets difficult. [4,6]

That baseline makes it easier to notice tension sooner and recover faster when stress shows up. A useful morning baseline is not a perfect meditation session. It is a few predictable cues that signal release: a longer exhale, a soft tongue posture, relaxed shoulders, and a neutral jaw with lips together and teeth apart. Small inputs early can reduce the need for constant correction later.[6,11]

The anchor

While your coffee is brewing or while brushing your teeth.

The practice: Vertical Expansion

Gently lift the sternum to open the chest.

Place the tongue on the palate just behind the upper front teeth.

235

Take three slow nasal breaths, focusing on the ribs expanding sideways rather than the chest lifting upward.

Why this works

This combination aligns posture, stabilizes the jaw without clenching, and signals safety to the nervous system. It sets a calm baseline for the trigeminal motor system so later demands require less bracing.

The Workday Practice

During the workday, jaw tension is most often driven by sustained focus, screen posture, and subtle breath holding. These inputs rarely feel dramatic in the moment. They build quietly, minute by minute, raising baseline muscle tone until clenching becomes the default response to concentration. [5,11]

Many people do not notice it until their teeth feel sore, their temples ache, or their neck feels tight. The objective in this chapter is not deep relaxation at your desk. It is mobility and regulation through frequent, light resets. Small adjustments performed often are more realistic than long breaks performed rarely. [2,6]

A 10-second reset at transitions can interrupt bracing before it consolidates: exhale slowly, let the tongue rest up, drop the shoulders, and re-check "lips together, teeth apart." When these micro-resets are stacked into routines you already do, they become automatic. The system stays fluid, tension clears before it accumulates, and the jaw stops carrying the full load of the workday.[2,11]

The anchor

Every time you send an email, finish a task, or take a sip of water.

236

The practice: The Vagal Reset[10,9]

Use the ClenchAlert Active Guard during your first sixty minutes of deep work. Perform a two second exhale with a soft vocal sigh. Briefly soften your vision and notice the edges of the room.

Why this works

This interrupts focal bracing and restores rhythmic breathing. It prevents allostatic load from building quietly and reduces the likelihood of afternoon headaches or jaw fatigue.

The Evening Practice

Evening rituals shape what your nervous system carries into the night. If you move from a high-demand day straight into bed without decompression, the body often keeps its protective tone. That lingering activation can show up as jaw bracing, nocturnal clenching, or grinding, even if you are not aware of it. Sleep is not a clean reset when the system is still running hot.[4,13]

The goal of decompression before sleep is to reduce load, not to solve everything. Evening is not the time to analyze your day or "train" your way out of tension. It is the time to unload. Choose cues that signal closure: dimmer light, fewer screens, slower breathing, and a brief jaw and shoulder release.

Keep it simple and repeatable.[13,6] A short routine done consistently teaches your body that it is safe to power down. Over time, that

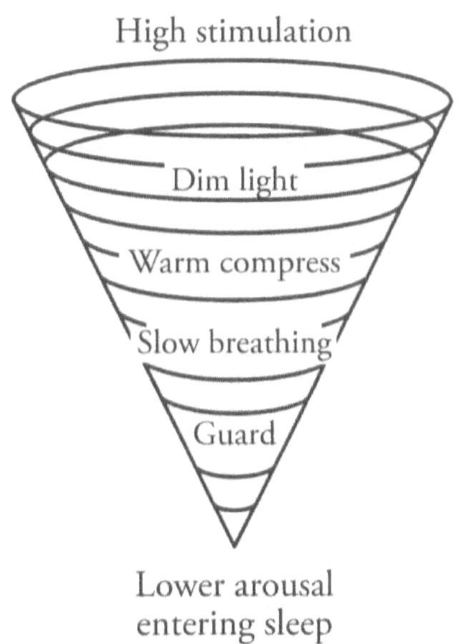

237

downshift often reduces nighttime bracing and improves morning recovery. The focus is not performance. It is creating conditions that make restoration more likely.[12,11]

The anchor

When you put your phone away for the night or after washing your face.

The practice: Sensory Unload[2,3]

Apply a warm compress to the jaw muscles for three minutes.

Insert your passive nighttime guard.

Practice 4-7-8 breathing. Inhale for four seconds, hold for seven, exhale for eight.

Why this works

Warmth increases blood flow and softens tissue. Slow breathing lowers cortisol and raises the arousal threshold. Together, these steps reduce micro arousals that trigger sleep related clenching.

Daily Routine Architecture

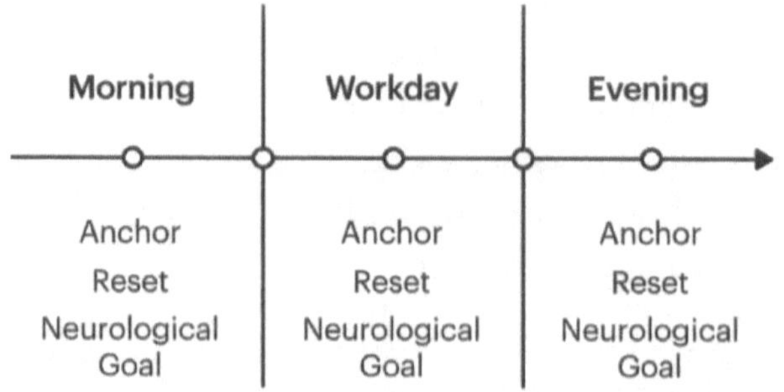

Building Your Personal Protocol

You do not need to overhaul your entire routine to change your jaw. In fact, trying to implement every ritual at once usually backfires. The nervous system does not learn through intensity. It learns through repetition.

Habits evolve best when they are simple, specific, and realistically paired with the life you already live.[2,3] Your goal is to build a personal protocol that fits your real schedule, not an idealized one. Think of it as designing a supportive rhythm rather than chasing a perfect day. Clenching thrives in chaos and urgency.

Regulation thrives in structure that feels doable.[4,2] Start by choosing three anchors you already perform without thinking: one in the morning, one during your workday, and one in the evening. Then attach a single jaw-supportive action to each anchor using the habit stacking formula:

After I do X, I will do Y. This is how you bypass willpower. The existing habit becomes the cue, and the new action becomes automatic over time.[3,2]

For the morning, pick an anchor that happens every day no matter what. Coffee brewing. Brushing your teeth. Feeding the dog. While that routine is already in motion, add one brief reset that establishes a calmer baseline. A sternum lift, tongue resting on the palate, and three nasal breaths can be enough.

The point is not to do a long practice. The point is to begin the day without armoring up.[6,11] For the workday, choose an anchor that repeats often. Sending an email. Joining a meeting. Taking a sip of water. These transitions are where tension accumulates.

Pair the anchor with a short vagal reset such as a soft exhale, a quick posture check, and a moment of peripheral softening. [6,2]

239

If you use ClenchAlert, this is also where it fits naturally: during your first focused block of work, it externalizes awareness so you are not spending your attention monitoring your jaw. When it vibrates, treat it as a neutral cue to reset, not a signal that you did something wrong.[10,9]

For the evening, select a shutdown cue that signals the day is complete. Putting your phone away. Washing your face. Changing into sleep clothes. Then add one decompression action that tells the nervous system it is safe to downshift.

Heat on the jaw for a few minutes, a short breathing pattern, and your passive guard if you need nighttime protection. This is how you reduce the echo of daytime stress that often shows up as nighttime clenching.[13,12]

Practice these three stacks consistently for two weeks before adding anything else. Two weeks gives your brain time to associate the new behavior with the old cue. It also allows you to notice what actually helps, which matters more than doing more.[2,3]

When regulation becomes rhythmic, clenching loses its job. Harmony is no longer something you chase. It becomes the default state your body can return to again and again.

If you would like, I can help you select a customized morning, workday, and evening stack based on your schedule, work demands, and known triggers.[1,4]

References

Habit Science, Automaticity, and Habit Stacking

1. Wood W, Rünger D. Psychology of habit. Annu Rev Psychol. 2016;67:289-314. doi:10.1146/annurev-psych-122414-033417

2. Lally P, van Jaarsveld CHM, Potts HWW, Wardle J. How are habits formed: modelling habit formation in the real world. Eur J Soc Psychol. 2010;40(6):998-1009. doi:10.1002/ejsp.674

3. Fogg BJ. Tiny Habits: The Small Changes That Change Everything. Houghton Mifflin Harcourt; 2019.

Stress Physiology, Allostatic Load, and Why Prevention Outperforms "Crisis Fixes"

4. McEwen BS. Protective and damaging effects of stress mediators. N Engl J Med. 1998;338(3):171-179. doi:10.1056/NEJM199801153380307

5. Arnsten AFT. Stress signalling pathways that impair prefrontal cortex structure and function. Nat Rev Neurosci.2009;10(6):410-422. doi:10.1038/nrn2648

Breathing as a Regulation Lever (Slow Breathing, Vagal Pathways, Downshift)

6. Lehrer PM, Gevirtz R. Heart rate variability biofeedback: how and why does it work? Front Psychol. 2014;5:756. doi:10.3389/fpsyg.2014.00756

7. Jerath R, Edry JW, Barnes VA, Jerath V. Physiology of long pranayamic breathing: neural respiratory elements may provide a mechanism that explains how slow deep breathing shifts the autonomic nervous system. Med Hypotheses. 2006;67(3):566-571. doi:10.1016/j.mehy.2006.02.042

Bruxism as Behavior; Biofeedback and Behavioral Approaches

8. Lobbezoo F, Ahlberg J, Raphael KG, et al. International consensus on the assessment of bruxism: report of a work in progress. J Oral Rehabil. 2018;45(11):837-844. doi:10.1111/joor.12663

9. de Albuquerque Vieira R, Oliveira-Souza AIS, Hahn L, Bähr S, Armijo-Olivo S, Ferreira PH. Effectiveness of biofeedback in individuals with awake bruxism compared to other types of treatment: a systematic review. Int J Environ Res Public Health. 2023;20(2):1558. doi:10.3390/ijerph20021558

10. Schwartz MS, Andrasik F, eds. Biofeedback: A Practitioner's Guide. 4th ed. Guilford Press; 2017.

Self-Management and Conservative Home Strategies (Warmth/Heat, Routine-Based Downshift)

11. Okeson JP. Management of Temporomandibular Disorders and Occlusion. 8th ed. Elsevier; 2019.

12. Nadler SF, Weingand K, Kruse RJ. The physiologic basis and clinical applications of cryotherapy and thermotherapy for the pain practitioner. Pain Physician. 2004;7(3):395-399.

13. Irish LA, Kline CE, Gunn HE, Buysse DJ, Hall MH. The role of sleep hygiene in promoting public health: a review of empirical evidence. Sleep Med Rev. 2015;22:23-36. doi:10.1016/j.smrv.2014.10.001

Chapter 16: The Body as Ongoing Feedback

If you want lasting change, you eventually have to move beyond managing symptoms and into relationship. Not a relationship with a device, a routine, or a set of rules, but a relationship with your own nervous system.

Most people start this work in a "monitor and correct" mindset. They check for clenching. They catch it. They stop it. They try again. That approach can create progress, but it is not sustainable as a long-term strategy because it relies on willpower. Willpower is finite. It fatigues. It collapses under pressure.

From monitoring and correcting to listening and responding.

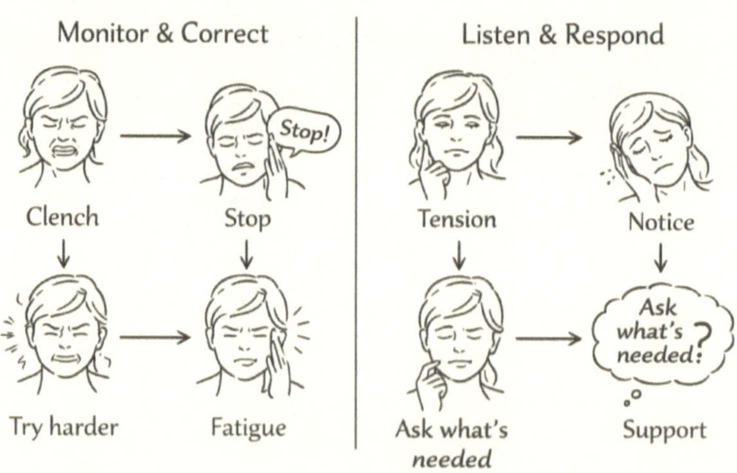

The long-term path is different. It is a shift from monitoring and correcting to listening and responding. This is interoception: the ability to sense the internal state of your body and interpret it as useful information. Interoception changes the meaning of jaw tension.

Instead of treating clenching as a failure or a defect, you begin to treat it as a signal. Your jaw becomes a dashboard. It reports on your internal environment in real time, including stress load, cognitive overload, emotional suppression, dehydration, fatigue, posture strain, and the need for boundaries. When you read the dashboard accurately, you stop fighting your body and start partnering with it.

This chapter is about building that partnership.

Cultivating the Body Trust Loop

Ongoing connection requires one foundational shift: you must stop treating body signals as betrayal. If clenching feels like your body is sabotaging you, you will naturally disconnect.

Disconnection is protective. It keeps you from feeling frustrated or disappointed. The problem is that disconnection also keeps you from receiving the early warnings that could prevent escalation.

The body trust loop starts with a new interpretation.

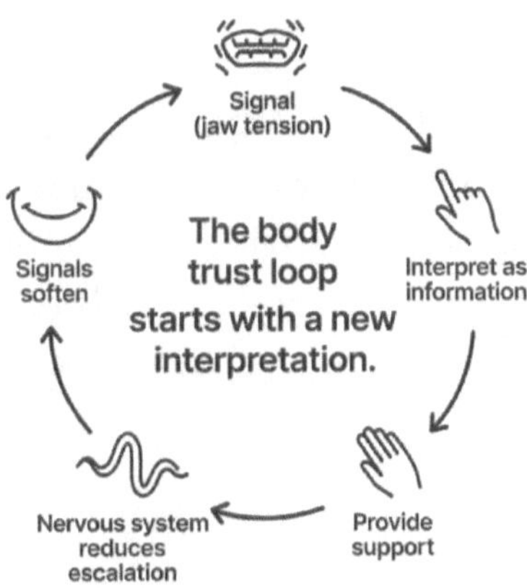

The interoceptive shift

When you feel tension, treat it as your body saying: "Something here requires our attention." This is not a slogan. It is a neurological reframe. When you interpret tension as information instead of failure, you reduce the threat response. That single change lowers the need for the body to escalate.

Then comes the most important part.

The responsive action

Instead of only stopping the clench, ask a better question: "What do I need right now?" Not what should I do. Not what is wrong with me. Not why can't I stop. A simple needs-based question. Possible answers are often practical and immediate:

- Water or electrolytes
- A two-minute break
- A posture reset or a short walk
- A boundary, such as pausing a task or delaying a response
- Food, sleep, or reduced stimulation
- A breath reset, such as a longer exhale

The result

When you respond to the signal with a real solution, your nervous system learns something essential: it does not have to scream to be heard. This is how internal trust forms. The body reduces the intensity of its signals when the signals reliably lead to support. Over time, the jaw stops escalating tension because escalation is no longer required.

The Soft Scan

A Lifelong Practice for Staying Online

As clenching becomes habitual, another problem often appears: sensory motor amnesia.[2,3,4] The jaw can be active for hours and still feel normal. The brain filters the tension out as background noise. That is why many people say, "I had no idea I was clenching until the headache started." To maintain long-term awareness, you need a simple practice that keeps the internal map sharp.

The practice

Three times a day, perform a ten-second Soft Scan. Do it during transitions, not as a formal "exercise," because transitions are when habits reset most easily.

The scan has three checkpoints:

Eyes: Are they hard or soft?

Tongue: Is it floating or pressed?

Pelvis: Are you gripping your seat or resting into it?

This is a scan, not a correction. The goal is to notice, not fix.

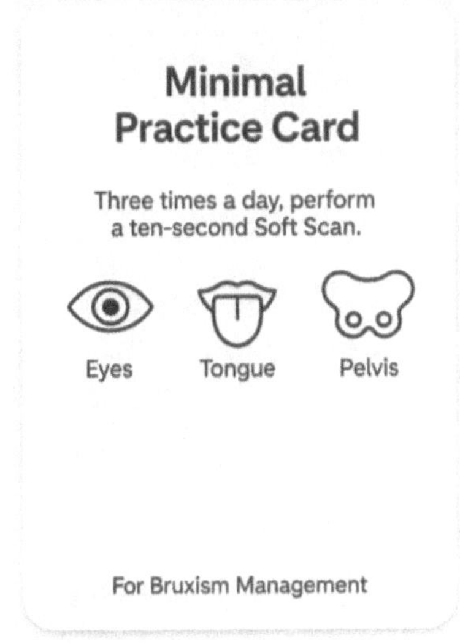

Why it works

A ten-second scan prevents the brain from filtering your jaw and posture out as noise. It keeps your somatosensory cortex, your internal body map, clear and updated. When your internal map stays detailed, you catch tension earlier. Early detection reduces intensity, reduces pain, and reduces the need for protective bracing. This is one of the most important long-term skills in the entire system. It makes your body easier to read and easier to regulate.

Using Biofeedback as a Tuning Fork

Biofeedback tools can accelerate learning because they provide an objective signal when awareness is still developing. The key, long term, is to shift how you relate to them. The goal is not to wear a tool forever because you cannot trust yourself. The goal is to use it to sharpen the skill of interoception so you can trust yourself more. This is why it helps to think of biofeedback as a tuning fork.

A tuning fork does not play the music for you. It gives you a reference note. It helps you calibrate.

The goal

Use your ClenchAlert periodically, perhaps one day a week, even after you feel significantly improved.

The purpose

It provides a standard of truth. It helps you recalibrate your internal sense of relaxed versus braced, especially if your baseline has slowly crept upward without you noticing. That slow creep is common. Stressful seasons happen. Posture slips. Sleep changes. Travel disrupts routine. Your jaw adapts quietly. A periodic tuning session brings your baseline back into alignment before clenching becomes loud again. This is how tools support independence rather than dependency.

Replacing Should, with Notice

Language is not just psychological. It is biological. In CBT, the word should tends to trigger a threat response. It implies that you are failing at something you are supposed to be doing. That subtle internal pressure matters because pressure is one of the nervous system's fastest triggers for bracing.

This is why the simplest long-term upgrade is linguistic. Old thought: "I should be relaxed right now." This often creates judgment, urgency, and muscle tone. New thought: "I notice my breathing is shallow and my jaw is active." This creates observation, space, and choice.

Neutral observation activates the prefrontal cortex, which has inhibitory connections to the amygdala. When the brain shifts from judgment to noticing, muscle tone often drops on its own. You create an internal environment where release becomes possible. Notice also preserves dignity. It keeps you in partnership rather than conflict.

Summary

The Long-Term Interoception Strategy

Skill	Daily Action	Long-Term Benefit
Validation	Acknowledge the clench as protective	Ends the internal war and lowers stress
Micro-resets	Ten-second Soft Scans during transitions	Keeps the internal map clear and active
Recalibration	Periodic use of Active Guard biofeedback	Prevents gradual return of unconscious clenching
Compassion	Replace judgment with curiosity	Maintains a parasympathetic baseline

The Body Wisdom Identity

The final shift is not a new technique. It is identity. If you see yourself as someone with a jaw problem, your attention naturally turns toward fixing. Fixing sounds practical, but it usually carries an invisible message: something is wrong and it needs to be corrected quickly. That urgency creates pressure. Pressure tells the nervous system that there is a problem to solve right now. And when the brain perceives urgency, it increases muscle tone. The jaw responds the way it always has, by bracing.

This is why many people get stuck in a frustrating loop. They notice clenching and immediately try to force it to stop. They monitor constantly, judge themselves for every slip, and treat tension as proof they are failing. Even if the intention is positive, the internal tone becomes corrective and harsh.

The body hears that tone as threat. The jaw tightens to meet it. The Body Wisdom Identity offers a different path. When you adopt the identity of a responsive body partner, your job is no longer to win a battle against tension. Your job is to listen, notice patterns, and respond skillfully. You treat jaw tension as information, not as a personal flaw. You do not demand perfection from your nervous system. You build a relationship with it.

This identity changes what you do in the moment. When you catch tension, you do not ask, "What is wrong with me?" You ask, "What is my system responding to?" You check the basics: breath, posture, hydration, workload, emotional strain, sleep debt. You make a small adjustment before the tension escalates. A longer exhale. A sternum lift. A softening of the eyes and tongue. A sip of water. A two minute reset between tasks. A boundary where you usually push through.

Over time, the nervous system learns something important: it does not have to shout to be heard. When you respond to early signals, the body stops needing stronger signals. Clenching begins to lose its role as the emergency broadcast system.

This is also where the BRUX Method becomes more than a framework. It becomes a way of living inside your day. You build awareness instead of waiting for pain. You relax intentionally instead of forcing release.

You understand triggers instead of blaming yourself. You exchange patterns instead of returning to old reflexes. Each repetition

251

strengthens the identity of someone who knows how to work with their body, not against it.

This attunement does not only protect your jaw. It protects your energy, because you stop spending it on constant bracing. It protects your sleep, because you reduce the stress that echoes into the night. It protects your mood, because self-criticism is replaced by curiosity and care. It protects your long-term health, because you become responsive to your own needs before the body has to break down to get your attention. Your jaw becomes a faithful messenger instead of an enemy. And your body becomes a place you can trust to tell you the truth.

References

Interoception, Body Awareness, and Internal State Monitoring

These sources support the core premise that jaw tension is an interoceptive signal, not a defect, and that sensing internal states improves regulation.

1. Khalsa SS, Adolphs R, Cameron OG, et al. Interoception and mental health: a roadmap. Biol Psychiatry Cogn Neurosci Neuroimaging. 2018;3(6):501-513. doi:10.1016/j.bpsc.2018.04.007

2. Craig AD. How do you feel? Interoception: the sense of the physiological condition of the body. Nat Rev Neurosci.2002;3(8):655-666. doi:10.1038/nrn894

3. Mehling WE, Price C, Daubenmier JJ, Acree M, Bartmess E, Stewart A. The Multidimensional Assessment of Interoceptive Awareness (MAIA). PLoS One. 2012;7(11):e48230. doi:10.1371/journal.pone.0048230

Habit Formation, Automaticity, and Sensory Filtering

These references support habit persistence, sensory-motor "tuning out," and why clenching can occur without conscious awareness.

4. Wood W, Rünger D. Psychology of habit. Annu Rev Psychol. 2016;67:289-314. doi:10.1146/annurev-psych-122414-033417

5. Graybiel AM. Habits, rituals, and the evaluative brain. Annu Rev Neurosci. 2008;31:359-387. doi:10.1146/annurev.neuro.29.051605.112851

6. Flor H, Diers M. Sensorimotor retraining and cortical reorganization in chronic pain. Handb Clin

Neurol.2013;116:403-412. doi:10.1016/B978-0-444-53497-2.00033-6

Biofeedback, Learning Loops, and Calibration

These sources support biofeedback as a learning accelerator and recalibration tool rather than a lifelong crutch.

7. Schwartz MS, Andrasik F, eds. Biofeedback: A Practitioner's Guide. 4th ed. Guilford Press; 2017.

8. Sato M, Iizuka T, Watanabe A, et al. EMG biofeedback training for daytime clenching behavior. J Oral Rehabil.2015;42(6):417-425. doi:10.1111/joor.12265

Cognitive Appraisal, Language, and Threat Physiology (CBT)

These references support the claim that judgmental language ("should") increases threat physiology, while neutral noticing supports regulation.

9. Beck JS. Cognitive Behavior Therapy: Basics and Beyond. 2nd ed. Guilford Press; 2011.

10. Ochsner KN, Gross JJ. The cognitive control of emotion. Trends Cogn Sci. 2005;9(5):242-249. doi:10.1016/j.tics.2005.03.010

Compassion, Safety Signaling, and Nervous System Learning

These sources support the role of compassion, safety cues, and reduced self-attack in lowering arousal and improving learning.

11. Gilbert P. The evolution of compassion and the implications for psychotherapy. Br J Clin Psychol. 2014;53(1):6-22. doi:10.1111/bjc.12036

12. Porges SW. The polyvagal theory: new insights into adaptive
    reactions of the autonomic nervous system. Cleve Clin J
    Med. 2009;76(Suppl 2):S86-S90. doi:10.3949/ccjm.76.s2.17

Epilogue: Awareness Is Medicine, and BRUX Is the Way You Practice It

If you take one idea from everything you have read, let it be this: awareness is not a passive observation. It is an active form of medicine. The moment you notice tension, change has already begun, because the nervous system cannot keep running the same program once attention is on it. Clenching thrives in the dark. BRUX is what you do the instant the lights come on.

That is why the goal was never perfection. It was never "never clench again." The goal was to build a reliable pathway back to neutral, back to safety, back to choice. This is what the BRUX Method is for. It is not a motivational slogan. It is a practical operating system for a protective nervous system.

Your jaw has never been trying to sabotage you. It has been trying to support you. It braces when your brain predicts demand, conflict, urgency, or threat. It clenches when your body believes it needs stability. It tightens when your emotions have no clean exit, when your posture asks your muscles to do the job your structure should be doing, when screens and deadlines keep your attention narrow, when sleep is disrupted and your arousal threshold is low, when pain convinces your brain that more guarding is the safest solution.

In every case, clenching is a strategy. It may be costly, but it is not random.

BRUX gives you a better strategy.

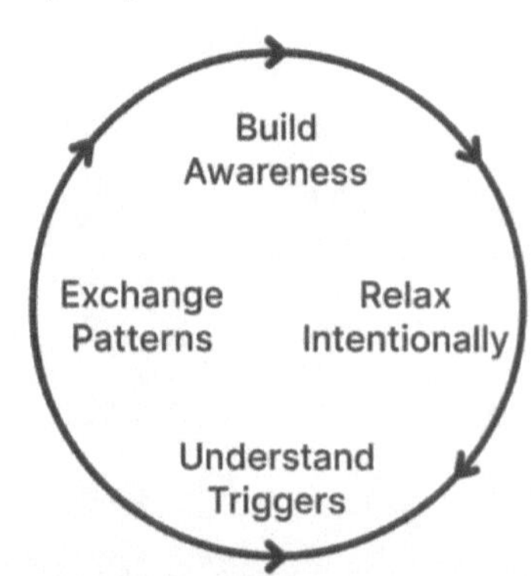

Build Awareness.

This is where healing starts. Not when you fix your bite. Not when you buy a tool. Not when you swear off stress. It starts when you catch the moment of pressure. The second your teeth touch, the second your tongue presses, the second your breath goes shallow, you are no longer trapped in an unconscious loop. You are in the first stage of change. Awareness is the interruption.

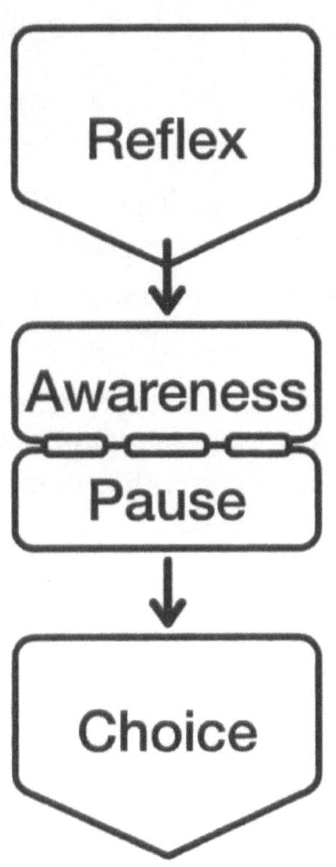

Awareness is the opening. Awareness is the hinge that turns a reflex into a choice. This is also why relapse is not a failure. It is information. It is simply awareness arriving later than you wanted. If you used to clench for hours and now you notice it in minutes, you are progressing.

If you used to wake up with pain and now you catch the tension the night before, you are progressing. The nervous system learns through repetition, but it also learns through timing. Faster noticing is a measurable win.

Relax Intentionally.

Not by forcing, not by fighting, and not by trying to "make" your jaw let go through effort. Relaxation is not a command. It is a condition. You create that condition by giving your nervous system signals of safety: a longer exhale, a softer gaze, warmth on the masseters, humming, stillness, slower transitions, posture that stacks the head

257

over the spine, hydration that keeps tissues pliable, routines that lower your allostatic load, sleep rhythms that reduce micro arousals.

Relaxation becomes available when safety is believable. This is why the method emphasizes softness. Your jaw does not release because you yelled at it. It releases because your body stops broadcasting threat. When you practice relax intentionally, you are not "being good." You are giving your biology what it needs to stop guarding.

Understand Triggers.

If awareness is the medicine, triggers are the diagnosis. Triggers are not just events. They are patterns: focused work, conflict avoidance, perfectionism, suppressed anger, sensory overload, forward head posture, shallow breathing, dehydration, hormonal shifts, fragmented sleep, nighttime arousals, airway instability. Most people keep trying to treat clenching at the level of the jaw, when clenching often begins upstream in the brain, the breath, the posture, the schedule, or the emotional load.

Understanding triggers is what makes your progress sustainable. Without it, you keep treating symptoms. With it, you redesign your environment. You stop asking, "What is wrong with my jaw?" and start asking, "What is my nervous system responding to, and what would help it feel safe right now?"

Exchange Patterns.

This is the part that turns BRUX into a lifestyle, not a project. You cannot delete a habit. You replace it. The old pathway may remain, but it no longer has to be the default. Exchange patterns means you do not just stop clenching. You substitute a new response that meets the same underlying need for stability, control, or protection, without the cost.

o Instead of clenching, you lengthen your exhale.

o Instead of bracing, you lift the sternum and stack the head.

o Instead of holding emotions in your jaw, you name them with compassion.

o Instead of scrolling late and sleeping lightly, you protect the wind down.

o Instead of fighting pain, you interrupt the pain-tension loop with safety signals.

o Instead of self-criticism, you choose curiosity and skillful adjustment.

o Instead of "powering through," you build rituals that keep your baseline low.

This is how harmony is built. Not through a single breakthrough, but through repeated exchanges that teach the nervous system a new default.

Where biofeedback fits and why it accelerates BRUX.

For many people, the hardest part of changing a jaw habit is not knowing you are doing it. That is the gap biofeedback closes. ClenchAlert is designed to turn unconscious daytime clenching into immediate, usable information by detecting bite pressure and delivering a gentle vibration cue in real time. It does not "fix" you and it is not meant to punish you. It acts like an external mirror:

clench, cue, reset.

259

Each cue becomes a clean rep of the BRUX Method. You build awareness the moment it vibrates. You relax intentionally with a simple posture and breath reset. You understand triggers by noticing what you were doing, thinking, or feeling when it happened.

You exchange patterns by choosing a softer response and returning to "lips together, teeth apart." Used this way, ClenchAlert is not a crutch. It is a training tool that helps your nervous system learn faster, because it reduces the time between the habit and the moment you can respond.

And then, quietly, something shifts.

You begin to notice earlier.
You reset faster.
Your body trusts you more.
Your jaw no longer has to shout to be heard.

At some point, you may realize the biggest change is not that you clench less. It is that you fear it less. You stop treating tension as proof that you are broken. You treat it as a signal that you are human and under load, and you know what to do next.

That is a profound kind of freedom.

This is the deeper promise of the BRUX Method. It is not just jaw relief. It is a new relationship with your internal world. A relationship where your body is not an enemy, not a problem to solve, and not a machine you must control. It is an intelligent system that communicates through sensation. When you learn its language, you do not need constant discipline. You need responsiveness.

So if you finish this and you still clench sometimes, that does not mean it did not work. It means you are alive. It means you have a nervous system that still tries to protect you under pressure. The question is no longer whether clenching will ever happen again. The question is what happens next.

Do you punish yourself, tighten more, and spiral into the old loop? Or do you practice BRUX?

Build awareness: "I notice I am bracing." Relax intentionally: "Let me make safety believable." Understand triggers: "What is driving this right now?" Exchange patterns: "What response would serve me better?"

That sequence is your way home.

In time, the jaw becomes what it was always meant to be: not a battlefield, but a barometer. A dashboard. A feedback system that keeps you honest about your stress, your posture, your sleep, your boundaries, your emotional truth. You stop chasing the fantasy of being tension free. You become skilled at returning to neutral.

And in that skill, you find the real outcome.

Not perfection.
Not control.
Harmony.

Because the minute you notice tension, change has already begun. BRUX is simply how you meet that moment, again and again, until awareness becomes familiar, safety becomes believable, and your jaw no longer needs to hold what your life can finally process.

Acknowledgments

This work stands on the shoulders of many disciplines, clinicians, researchers, and lived experiences that have shaped how we understand bruxism, pain, and nervous system regulation.

I want to acknowledge the clinicians and researchers in sleep diagnostics and sleep therapy whose work has made invisible physiology measurable and treatable. Their commitment to objective data, longitudinal follow-up, and patient-centered care transformed sleep from a vague complaint into a clinical science. Their work continues to remind us that airway, arousal, oxygenation, and nervous system load are inseparable from jaw health.

I am deeply indebted to the pioneers of cognitive behavioral therapy and habit science, whose frameworks clarified that change is not a matter of willpower, but of learning, context, and repetition. Their contributions reframed relapse as information, behavior as adaptive, and compassion as a prerequisite for lasting change.

This work is also informed by leaders in neurological retraining, biofeedback, and interoception, who helped articulate how awareness, feedback, and bodily sensing can gently reshape automatic patterns. Their research demonstrated that the nervous system learns best through safety, precision, and repetition rather than force.

On a personal level, I owe profound gratitude to the clinicians who mentored me and shaped my thinking long before *The BRUX Method* had a name.

Dr. L. Wayne Halstrom taught me the power of patient mentorship. His clinical example inspired my dedication to oral appliance therapy for the treatment of obstructive sleep apnea and reinforced the idea that technical skill means little without deep responsibility to the person wearing the device.

Dr. Edward Spiegel introduced me to alternative approaches to head, neck, and facial pain decades before orofacial pain became a recognized specialty. His work challenged rigid thinking and planted the early seeds of a systems-based view of pain that still informs my work today.

Dr. John Viviano impressed upon me the value of a literature-based approach to sleep and pain therapy. From him, I learned that innovation without evidence is fragile, and that careful reading, skepticism, and clinical humility are essential to serving patients well.

Dr. Bradley Eli has consistently thought outside the box and generously served as a sounding board for new ideas. His willingness to question assumptions and explore unconventional connections created a safe space for intellectual incubation and clinical growth.

Finally, **Jim Glidewell**, CDT, taught me that constant change is not something to fear, but something to expect, encourage, and embrace. His philosophy reinforced that progress in healthcare requires adaptability, curiosity, and the courage to rethink established norms.

Most importantly, I want to recognize the patients. Those who wake with sore jaws, headaches, and fatigue. Those who have tried to "just relax" and blamed themselves when it did not work. Your persistence, curiosity, and willingness to understand your body more deeply are the true reason this work exists. Your search for relief is not weakness. It is wisdom.

Author's Note
On integrating science, compassion, and real-world practice to create a realistic path toward everyday calm.